Dieting
IN REAL LIFE

*101 Tips and Inspiration
for a Healthier You*

JUGGLING
OUR LIVES

ELLYN SANNA

BARBOUR BOOKS
An Imprint of Barbour Publishing, Inc.

Published by Barbour Books, an imprint of Barbour Publishing, Inc., P.O. Box 719, Uhrichsville, Ohio 44683
www.barbourbooks.com

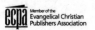 Member of the
Evangelical Christian
Publishers Association

Contents

INTRODUCTION

As women, we are constantly bombarded with the message that we need to lose weight. The message comes at us from all directions, in several forms.

First, our culture tells us that each and every one of us needs to look like a Barbie doll, with long, slender legs and a narrow waist. Advertising, movies, and television seldom allow for different kinds of beauty; instead, the implication is that only one kind of body is acceptable. What's worse is the underlying message that we are somehow not worth as much as women if we do not conform to the Barbie-doll cookie-cutter shape.

We may try to divorce ourselves from the world's standards for beauty—but it's harder to argue with the constant warnings from the medical community about the dangers of being overweight. Carrying too much fat on our bodies is not good for our circulatory systems. We would all live longer and feel healthier and stronger if we were not overweight.

Last of all comes the "Christian message": Gluttony—overeating—is a sin. The apostle Paul advises us to do all things in moderation. We are not to make food our idol.

With all these voices speaking the same message, it's no wonder that a study of a thousand women found that losing weight was the most common goal shared by all the group members. After all, how can we be complacent about our weight when we have so many reasons for feeling ashamed of it?

Sooner or later most of us who could stand to lose ten or fifteen pounds (or five—or fifty) try to do something about it. When we do, we find there are even more voices out there offering solutions to our condition. Any women's magazine we pick up has at least one article about weight loss. Diet books are best-sellers. Everywhere we turn we find another diet plan that promises to work miracles.

And so we try these various diets. Some of us may lose the weight we had hoped to—while others of us may become frustrated and give up before we see any success at all. Either way, sooner or later, most of us go back to eating the way we always did. If our weight does go down, eventually it creeps right back to where it was before—or even higher.

Placed then amid these temptations,
I strive daily against sin in eating and drinking.
For it is not of such nature that I can
settle on cutting it off once for all,
and never touching it afterward.

AUGUSTINE

That's the thing about eating—you can't just go cold turkey and "cut it off once for all," as Augustine says. Eventually, you have to eat. To give up eating altogether would be far more destructive than overeating, and eating disorders like anorexia are dangerous diseases that are all too common, particularly among young women. Instead, somehow we have to learn how to practice moderation. Instead of "going on a diet," we have to find new ways to think about food and eating.

NO TIME TO DIET

But our lives are already so full of other responsibilities. As women, we're often busy from morning 'til night taking care of our families. Every day we juggle a hundred different responsibilities:

careers, laundry, friendships, spending time with our children, feeding our families, housework, being daughters, being wives, church work, other volunteer work, yard work, correspondence, bills. . . . The list goes on and on and on.

We're scrambling so fast to keep all these different "balls" up in the air that we seldom have time to take care of ourselves—so all too often we let the "ball" that consists of diet and exercise bounce off into the corner. There it sits, neglected, gathering dust, a source of guilt whenever we glance at it. One day, we tell ourselves, when we're not so busy. . .when the kids are in school. . .when we get this project done. . . when we feel better physically. . .when life is ideal. Of course that never happens.

Conditions are never just right.
People who delay action until all
factors are favorable
are the kind who do nothing.

WILLIAM FEATHER

A WOMAN'S JUGGLING ACT

For several years now I've been talking and writing about juggling as a metaphor for our lives as women. At first, the juggling image seemed to me to be merely a description of the frustration I felt with my life: If I did one thing, then I didn't have time to do something else.

For instance, if I took time to exercise every day, I soon found that the dirty clothes in my laundry room had accumulated in a mound roughly the same height as my youngest child. When I sat in front of the computer pursuing my career as an editor and writer, I neglected to create healthy, nonfattening meals; instead, I tended to grab a doughnut for breakfast, a peanut butter sandwich for lunch, and order a pizza for supper. When I went for long, brisk walks, my children felt neglected. If I went on a low-carbohydrate diet, my husband complained that I wasn't cooking pasta often enough. I could never seem to do everything and please everybody at the same time. I couldn't possibly keep all the "balls" up in the air.

I put a lot of attention into taking care of my family, but all too often I simply gave up trying to take care of myself. Instead, I satisfied myself with those doughnuts, peanut butter sandwiches, and pizza, because, after all, they tasted good. Juggling the pieces of my life as fast as I could, I felt I at least deserved to eat what I wanted. The juggling metaphor was merely a word picture for my frustration.

When I researched juggling as an actual physical activity, however, I was surprised to find that the metaphor actually offers us hope. A juggler, I discovered, is someone who creates a pattern out of many separate pieces; a juggler spins everything together into one, unified whole.

As a follower of Christ, I find that He is the One who makes sense out of all the pieces of my life; He is the pattern that pulls everything else together. If everything I do—whether it's writing a book or cleaning a toilet—is offered up to Him, then all of it, all the spinning pieces I juggle, becomes valuable and significant. At the same time, no individual responsibility weighs as much when I toss it up into Christ's hands—and if my one goal is to serve Him, then it really doesn't matter if I end up dropping a few balls. The only thing that matters is that I keep my focus on Jesus. He will work out the timing.

To every thing there is a season,
and a time to every purpose under the heaven.

ECCLESIASTES 3:1 KJV

JUGGLING WITH JESUS

We do not juggle alone, for Jesus is with us. If we keep Him at the center of our juggling acts, then He will not only help us to juggle more smoothly, but He will also give us wisdom to know which balls He wants us to pick up and which ones He wants us to drop for now (or forever).

As women, most of us have learned to always put ourselves last. It just seems to come with the territory. We may resent doing this, but we still believe it's what all good women have to do. We even assume that God must approve of our unselfish behavior. But the truth is, God doesn't put a woman's needs last.

When God looks at our families, He doesn't see that everyone deserves time and attention except the women. Instead, He loves and treasures each of us—including the women in the family. He wants to bless us all. And He knows that as women we can't keep on meeting all our responsibilities indefinitely if we never take care of ourselves. He doesn't want the whole family to be nourished and cared for while we women are emotionally and spiritually—and sometimes physically—undernourished. He wants to sustain us all—and He wants to help us women take better care of ourselves.

There is much food here for those
who know how to digest it.
May the Holy Ghost lead us
into its marrow and fatness!

CHARLES SPURGEON

TAKING TIME TO HEAR GOD'S VOICE

As a mother, as a professional person, as a wife and a friend and a daughter and a church volunteer, I often get confused by all the conflicting messages I hear. Everyone wants something different from me. And I seldom hear anyone telling me to take care of myself. Of course I also hear the messages that tell me to lose weight, but they only make me feel guilty. I'm so busy responding to all the other voices, I simply don't have the energy left to consistently do anything about my physical condition.

That's why I need to make a regular time in my schedule when I sit down in God's presence and reevaluate my life. I need to draw away for at least a brief time from all the other voices and find out what God wants me to include in my juggling routine. Which "balls" does He want me to be juggling? How can I do that more efficiently? (For more specific help with time management, see another Juggling Our Lives book, *Balance for Busy Moms*.) I find that if I spend one hour a week prayerfully considering the various pieces of my life, I juggle more smoothly throughout the week. I'm less apt to get confused about what God wants for me. I'm not as likely to go lunging off in all directions, trying to please the loudest voices I hear.

That doesn't mean I don't need to daily make time for God in my life, as well. When I have no small quiet space alone with Him throughout my day, I tend to find my juggling act overwhelming and exhausting. Even more, I find that juggling becomes a joy when I consciously, moment by moment, toss each "ball" into God's waiting hands, trusting Him for the tiniest details. But a weekly "planning session" with God helps me keep my daily time with

Him more focused, even as I work to practice living in His presence moment by moment.

These once-a-week sessions with Jesus are a good time for me to give my life a closer look. What's working? What isn't? Which "balls" am I neglecting that God wants me to pick up off the floor? Which should I set down to make room for these new activities?

If we make a regular time to ask God for His insights on our life, I suspect that many of us would find He wants us to begin taking better care of ourselves. We don't have to wait for someone else to do it for us; this is something we can do for ourselves. And we don't have to wait for a better time when things are less busy or we're feeling stronger. We don't have to wait for anything. With God's help, we can begin right now to take care of ourselves spiritually, emotionally, physically.

Do what you can, with what
you have, where you are.

THEODORE ROOSEVELT

We cannot do everything at once,
but we can do something at once.

CALVIN COOLIDGE

PAYING ATTENTION TO OUR DIETS

We're used to connecting diets with deprivation. Although most of us would like to be thinner, we don't see weight loss as a way to do something nice for ourselves. It's just too hard.

But the truth is, dropping pounds is not the impossible task we sometimes make it out to be. With God's help, this is something we *can* do, no matter how weak our willpower and personal strength. We read in 2 Corinthians 12:9 and 10 that when "I am weak, then am I strong," for God's "strength is made perfect in weakness." As we let go of our lives (including our diets and exercise habits) and give them to God, we allow His strength to work miracles in our lives.

Paying attention to our diets is a way we can take better care of ourselves. We shouldn't look at it as a way to deprive ourselves, but as a wonderful gift we can give ourselves, a way to see that we're truly nourished.

"When you have eaten your fill,
praise the LORD your God for the
good. . .he has given you."

DEUTERONOMY 8:10 NLT

UNCONDITIONALLY LOVED

This book is not a diet or exercise plan, but it will give you practical tips for managing your weight. These are based on research, and they are all things I have found useful in my own life. I hope you, too, will find they work for you.

These tips are not, however, a set of rigid rules and demanding activities you have to somehow find the time to squeeze into your already busy life. Instead, they are meant to be gentle suggestions that will guide you toward developing a change in the way you think about diet, exercise, and your physical appearance. As your attitudes about these things grow healthier, more in line with what God wants for you, then you'll find you begin to change, both on the inside and the outside. Leave the degree and the speed of that change up to God. Focus on Him rather than on your weight.

And whether you lose weight or not, remember this: Jesus loves you just as much, no matter if you're a size 22 or a size 5. There is nothing you have to do to earn His love. He wants the best for each of us, and I suspect being physically healthy is a part of that "best."

You are already beautiful in His eyes. Right now, just the way you are at this moment, you are completely, unconditionally loved. You don't have to lose weight to prove your worth to Him. You are infinitely and uniquely precious.

So if you decide you want to lose weight, don't do it to win Jesus' approval. Instead, with His help, do it for yourself.

You are so beautiful, my beloved,
so perfect in every part.

SONG OF SONGS 4:7 NLT

CHAPTER 1
Changing Our Attitudes

1

*Don't let your physical appearance
define your identity:
There is more to you
than just your body.*

We live in a world where all too often we judge
each other by how closely our outward appearance conforms to the current fashion. We act as
though there were some absolute standard for
clothing, hair, and weight—but all you have to
do is walk through an art museum, and the
paintings from various eras will tell you this fact:
The human concept of what's beautiful in terms
of clothes, hairstyle, and body shape has changed
drastically from century to century. We twenty-
first-century women are embarrassed if we have

a plump, pear-shaped body—and yet that very same body would have been the epitome of feminine loveliness in an earlier era.

Don't let the world's passing fashions define your worth. We are eternal beings, inhabitants of God's everlasting kingdom. Our bodies are simply one aspect of who we are. They are a precious part of our identities, and they deserve our care— but who we really are, who we are in God's eyes, goes far beyond the world's fickle judgment of our external appearance.

When body and soul are finally
completely united, who can imagine the
glory they will possess? At last they will achieve
their full potential; they will be all
that God originally created them to be,
totally united, with no jarring division between
them so they can serve the Lord
with shouts of thanksgiving, a crown
of everlasting joy upon their head.

JOHN BUNYAN, *THE RICHES OF BUNYAN*

> The Spirit itself beareth
> witness with our spirit, that
> we are the children of God.
>
> ROMANS 8:16

2 Get your value from being a child of God—rather than from being successful at weight loss.

All of us need to feel a healthy sense of our own worth—but too often we try to derive our self-worth from sources that sooner or later let us down. If we count on our jobs or our relationships—or our weight-loss programs—to make us feel good about ourselves, then so long as we are experiencing success, we feel proud and full of self-esteem. But eventually, inevitably, we find that in one way or another we have failed. When that happens, if we have pinned all our hopes to these sources of self-worth, a terrible blow is struck to our identities.

Strict diet plans are a form of legalism—a

way to earn our worth by conforming to the letter of the law. The truth is, none of us, no matter how determined and self-disciplined we are, can keep all the rules all the time. This sets us up for repeated failures that lead to discouragement, guilt, and depression.

Don't focus all your energies on your weight-loss program. Jesus is the true source of your worth, and He is the one source that will never let you down. His love for you is eternal and unchanging. Once we begin to grasp that fact, our occasional lapses—and even our colossal failures—will no longer shake our sense of self-worth.

Because the creature itself
also shall be delivered
from the bondage of corruption
into the glorious liberty
of the children of God.

ROMANS 8:21 KJV

Diet **FACT**

Recent studies indicate that 97 million adult Americans can be classified as overweight or obese—and yet at the same time the diet industry is booming. If all these diet plans worked, why are there still so many overweight people in our country? One researcher found that of the approximately 26,000 diets that have been marketed, about 95 percent of them have failed to produce any significant weight loss.

> For what is enough for health, is too little
> for pleasure. . . . In this uncertainty the unhappy
> soul rejoiceth, and therein prepares an excuse
> to shield itself, glad. . .that under the cloak of
> health, it may disguise the matter of gratification.
> These temptations I daily endeavour to resist,
> and I call on Thy right hand, and to Thee
> do I refer my perplexities; because I have
> as yet no settled counsel herein.
>
> AUGUSTINE

3 Concentrate on being healthy rather than achieving a Barbie-doll figure.

A growing number of experts say the most important concept for good health is not fat but fit. When you set out to develop a more healthy lifestyle, you may lose weight in the process. If you do, fine. If you don't—well, then that's fine, too.

Still, it's hard to sort all the conflicting messages in our heads. Even Augustine, the great church father who lived centuries ago, struggled with this same dilemma: How do I determine the line between a healthy appetite and overeating?

I find, though, that my internal focus shapes my external behavior. When I stop obsessing over the fact that I'm not model-thin and instead seek to care for my body as best I can, then my eating habits no longer ride the seesaw between over-indulgence and starvation.

Ultimately, beauty comes in all different shapes and sizes. The important thing is to enjoy the sense of energy and well-being that a healthy lifestyle produces. We want to be all we can be, both for ourselves and for God's kingdom.

Seek ye first the kingdom of God. . .
and all these things shall be added unto you.

MATTHEW 6:33 KJV

 Diet FACT

Experts say that even a 5 to 10 percent reduction in total body weight can significantly improve risk factors for heart disease and diabetes, as well as reduce your odds for osteoarthritis. Even if you can't drop 5 percent of your weight, your health is likely to benefit from better eating and exercise habits.

4 Don't let past failures or the size of your goal discourage you.

The more weight we have to lose, the more difficult it often is to begin to change our eating
habits. I have the same reaction to almost any
task, whether it's cleaning my house or writing
a book: The more enormous the job looks, the
less likely I am to begin. Like the children of
Israel who put off entering the Promised Land,
I'm afraid of giants. And I'm even more afraid
to tackle a giant if I know he's conquered me in
the past. I'd rather not try at all than risk feeling like a failure yet again.

But God's not asking us to lose a hundred
pounds (or even five) right now, right this
minute. Instead, He's simply asking us to put
our hands in His and take one step. It may be a
tiny little step, like going for a walk after lunch
or saying no to a second helping at dinner. After

we make that step, another one will follow, and then another, each one small and manageable.

It's okay to glance up at our end goal now and then, just to make sure we're still on course. But we're less likely to become overwhelmed and discouraged when our attention is fixed on our journey's companion rather than the goal we hope to reach. He will give us the strength we need to face any giant. . .and He will lead us into the Promised Land.

What is important is to begin.

HUGH PRATHER

> Thou hast taught me, good Father,
> that to the pure, all things are pure;
> but that it is evil unto the man that eateth
> with offence; and, that every creature of Thine
> is good, and nothing to be refused, which
> is received with thanksgiving. . . These things
> have I learned, thanks be to Thee, praise
> to Thee, my God, my Master, knocking at
> my ears, enlightening my heart;
> deliver me out of all temptation.
>
> AUGUSTINE

5 Change your attitude toward food.

Sometimes I turn food into a god. When I'm sad and tired, I turn for comfort to a chocolate chip cookie (or two or three or. . .). And then there are those times when suddenly life seems dull and drab—and I reach for brownie fudge ice cream as the only thing that can restore my spirits. God may have some other blessing He was longing to give me in both these instances—but I chose to worship at my idol's feet instead.

31

Food can also be a cruel god. Our minds become so steeped in the "dieting mentality" that we feel virtuous when we nibble on a stick of celery and sinful when we indulge in a slice of birthday cake. We want to be "good"—and yet, oh, how we long for those forbidden delights. We find ourselves obsessing over food—and inevitably we yield to our cravings. When we do, we know we've fallen from righteousness; now we're "bad."

But we need to stop labeling foods "good" and "bad." Restricting favorite foods only leads to more cravings and eventually to overeating. Instead, we can with moderation include in our diets our favorite foods. Then our focus can be on healthful eating, not dieting. Food was meant to be a gift, not a god.

One must eat to live, not live to eat.

MOLIÈRE

Food does not bring us near to God;
we are no worse if we do not eat,
and no better if we do.

I CORINTHIANS 8:8

6

*Stop focusing only on your weight;
focus on the rest of what life
has to offer.*

In striving to reach my goal—the perfect body—
I sometimes miss out on what really matters.
Loving and working, playing and talking, praying
and dreaming—these are the important things
in life.

When I think about a time in my life when
I weighed less, I realize I wasn't any happier then
than I am now. No, my happiest moments are
when I sense God's presence or when I'm with
the people I love. The joy in those moments has
nothing to do with any diet plan.

Life, we learn too late,
is in the living, in the tissue
of every day and hour.

STEPHEN LEACOCK

7 Start living as if you were at your ideal weight right now.

Psychologists have found that people perform better and achieve more when they focus on the positive rather than the negative. That's why hating my body is not a good motivator for change. If I habitually think of myself as overweight, I tend to get discouraged and give up. My mental habit becomes a self-fulfilling prophecy.

But God wants me to be whole—emotionally, spiritually, and physically. Through Jesus, that wholeness is mine now, in the present moment. As I lay claim to God's wholeness spiritually and emotionally, I will be far more motivated to live it out in my body, as well.

After all, I am one being: body, mind, and soul. Sometimes I try to divide up those three aspects of my identity into separate neat packages. I assume I can hate my physical self while I accept Christ's salvation spiritually and emotionally.

But Jesus wants to heal all of me. He offers me health right now, this minute. I don't have to earn it by sticking to a strict diet and exercise program; I don't have to wait until I lose a certain amount of pounds. It's mine now.

Enter thou into the joy of thy lord.

MATTHEW 25:21 KJV

8 *Appreciate the gift God has given you: your body.*

Even if we are a little overweight—even if we are a *lot* overweight—our bodies are still amazing and miraculous. We may experience some physical limitations, but think of all we *can* do: We have the visual acuity to see a sunrise or a child's face. . .the power to communicate love and ideas. . .the sensitivity to feel the touch of a hand or a breeze against our faces. . .the mental strength to solve puzzles and create new concepts. . .muscles that move our hands to clasp and give and work. . . . Clearly, there is so much more to our bodies than just their weight.

When God designed the human body, His goal was perfection. No matter how much you weigh, don't be ashamed to enjoy this marvelous gift God has given you.

DIETING IN REAL LIFE

Is not sight a jewel?
Is not hearing a treasure?
Is not speech a glory?
O my Lord, pardon my ingratitude
and pity my dullness
who am not sensible of these gifts.

THOMAS TRAHERNE

I praise you because
I am fearfully and wonderfully made;
your works are wonderful,
I know that full well.

PSALM 139:14

9

*If you make mistakes and fall off
the wagon, don't wait until
tomorrow to start over.*

So many times I've started a diet plan, only to
yield to temptation after only a week or so of
effort. My impulse then is to simply give up.
With a sigh of relief, I reach for yet another
brownie. *I'll begin again,* I tell myself, *when conditions are more ideal: after the weekend. . .when
the summer's over. . .after the holidays. . . .* And
with that decision, I give myself permission to
overindulge once more.

But if I stop going "on a diet," I avoid this
pitfall. If instead I aim for a new way of living,
then when I overeat I can simply get myself back

on track as quickly as possible. Gradually, as I persist, I form new eating habits—and habits are far more effective than mere willpower.

In the meantime, I need to stop demanding perfection of myself. We all fall short of God's glory—but Jesus doesn't call me to be perfect; He only calls me to follow Him. Wallowing in guilt and despair is a waste of time when all the while Jesus is still calling me.

If you pigged out today, see what you can learn from the experience. And then begin again, right now. Each and every moment brings a new opportunity to start anew.

You may have to fight a battle
more than once to win it.

MARGARET THATCHER

Success is to be measured not
so much by the position
one has reached in life as by the obstacles
which he has overcome while trying to succeed.

BOOKER T. WASHINGTON

> Yet because I thought them to be Thee,
> I fed thereon; not eagerly, for Thou didst
> not in them taste to me as Thou art; for
> Thou wast not these emptinesses, nor was
> I nourished by them, but exhausted rather.
>
> AUGUSTINE

10 *If your extra weight is a symptom of some other problem, deal with that problem first.*

Centuries ago, Augustine understood the temptation to turn to food for nourishment, refreshment, and excitement. We often eat whenever we have a problem, whether it's physical, psychological, or spiritual. And overeating only makes our problems worse.

But losing weight isn't a magic answer, either. Excess weight can be a symptom of another physical problem. It can also be a symptom of emotional or spiritual distress. In those cases, no matter how much weight we lose, we will still be lacking true health. Our bodies, our hearts, or our souls will still be crying out for something more.

Sometimes it's easier to pin all our discomfort on one thing. *If I could only be thin,* we tell ourselves, *then I would feel better, then I'd be happy, then my life wouldn't seem so empty. . . .* But this is a false hope.

As we begin to think about our bodies in a new way, we often need help in seeing where our true strengths and weaknesses lie. We will need to talk to our doctors. . .our pastors. . .our friends who work together with us to be the Body of Christ. We may need to seek out a counselor. And we definitely need to open our hearts to God.

He wants to heal us wherever we are wounded. Let's not be so focused on our weight that we miss out on the full bounty of His healing love.

He forgives all my sins and heals all my diseases.

PSALM 103:3 NLT

But unto you that fear my name
shall the Sun of righteousness arise
with healing in his wings.

MALACHI 4:2 KJV

> We have to learn to be our own best friends
> because we fall too easily into the trap
> of being our worst enemies.
>
> RODERICK THORP

11

Be gentle with yourself: Support and encourage yourself, the way you would a friend or one of your children.

All too often we are harder on ourselves than anyone else. Listen to your silent internal dialogue sometime. . .for instance, the next time you're trying on a bathing suit in a store changing room. Now imagine a friend—or your daughter—was trying on a bathing suit. Would you brutally point out every bulge and dimple? Even if that particular bathing suit wasn't a good choice, wouldn't you still focus on the positive as much as possible? Wouldn't you temper your honesty with gentleness?

As women, most of us have learned the art of affirmation. Of course none of us are perfect at it, even with those we love the most; but still our goal is generally to build up our loved ones rather than to tear them down. We need to practice these same skills with ourselves.

Stop being so critical with yourself. The next time you feel upset about your weight, treat yourself as gently as you would an anxious child. Try demonstrating to yourself the love described in 1 Corinthians 13.

Love is patient, love is kind. . . .
It always protects. . .always hopes,
always perseveres.

1 CORINTHIANS 13:4, 7

Let your gentleness be evident to all.

PHILIPPIANS 4:5

> No sin is too big for God to pardon,
> and none too small for habit to magnify.
>
> B. Joseph Pakuda

12 *Forgive yourself.*

We have all made mistakes; some of these mistakes—like an overweight body—are more visible than others. But in God's eyes, those who are overweight are no worse than those who may have perfect bodies yet hide deep in their hearts their separation from God. All of us need God's healing grace.

We know that God wants us to forgive others, but we don't always extend the same gift to ourselves. And yet Jesus Christ has already offered us complete and total forgiveness. If we refuse to forgive ourselves, then we have trapped our hearts in a prison of our own making.

In reality, Christ has already flung open the door. All we have to do is walk free.

DIETING IN REAL LIFE

Forgiveness is the finding again
of a lost possession.

FRIEDRICH SCHILLER

In him we have redemption through his blood,
the forgiveness of sins,
in accordance with the riches of God's grace
that he lavished on us. . . .

EPHESIANS 1:7–8

Where is that foolish person
who thinks it in [her] power
to commit more than God could forgive?

FRANCIS DE SALES

> "Do not worry about for tomorrow;
> for tomorrow will care for itself."
>
> MATTHEW 6:34 NAS

13

Don't worry about how fast you lose weight; if you have reached a plateau phase or even if your weight goes up a little, do not despair.

When I step on the scales and see I've lost several pounds, a warm glow settles over me for the rest of the day. It's as though the scales sang out, "You are successful, you are worthy, you are good!" But by the same token, when I step on the scales and see I've put on a few pounds, a dark pall falls over my heart. This time I act as though the scales muttered, "You failed, you're ugly, you're *bad!*" And then I spend the rest of the day fretting about my weight, worrying that I'll never be able to lose those pounds.

How silly I am to give a set of bathroom

scales such power over my life! In effect, I'm worshiping at the feet of another god than the God of love who wants me whole. When instead my eyes are fixed on Him, I can trust Him to provide for me on my "diet journey"— today. . .and tomorrow. . .and forever. And then I can stop worrying so much about the ups and downs along the way.

Worry never robs tomorrow of its sorrow;
it only saps today of its strength.

A. J. CRONIN

> No one can make you feel inferior
> without your consent.
>
> ELEANOR ROOSEVELT

14 Refuse to listen to the world's propaganda about beauty.

Everywhere I turn I see and hear media messages that tell me how I ought to look: thin, long-legged, firm-skinned. It's so easy to measure myself against this standard for beauty—and when I do, I come up lacking.

How foolish I am, though, to look to the advertising industry for validation. Its purpose, after all, is not to affirm my appearance as it is but to convince me I *need* a particular product that will magically transform me.

I don't need to be a slave to changing fashion or self-serving advertising. Through Christ I am already transformed.

DIETING IN REAL LIFE

Fashion condemns us to many follies;
the greatest is to make oneself its slave.

NAPOLEON BONAPARTE

So we have stopped evaluating others
by what the world thinks about them. . . .
They are not the same anymore,
for. . .a new life has begun!

2 CORINTHIANS 5:16–17 NLT

To be nobody but yourself—in a world
which is doing its best, night and day,
to make you everybody else—means to fight
the hardest battle which any human can fight,
and never stop fighting.

E. E. CUMMINGS

15 *Find your happiness in the present moment, the here and now; don't wait to lose weight before you allow yourself to appreciate life's joy.*

If only I were married, I used to think back in my single days, *then I would be happier.* And then I fell in love and married, and yes, marriage was marvelous—but almost immediately I began to think, *If only we had our own house. . . .* And then it was, *If only we could have children. . .* and then, *If only I could achieve this professional goal. . . .* Lately, that interior voice has been whispering, *If only I could lose weight. . . .*

It's good to have goals; they help us find direction and keep our focus. But we need to understand that these goals cannot provide a true answer to our dissatisfaction with our lives or with ourselves. All too often, even as we reach some longed-for achievement, we find happiness receding in front of us, the way witch water does on hot pavement.

God wants you to find satisfaction in the life He's given you right now, this very minute. He wants you to find joy in being yourself, now, as you stand before Him. No matter how positive and constructive your goal may be, happiness is *now, here,* in the presence of the One who loves you.

Whenever you get there, there's no there there.

GERTRUDE STEIN

This is the day which the LORD hath made;
we will rejoice and be glad in it.

PSALM 118:24 KJV

> A [woman] too busy to take care
> of [her] health is like a mechanic
> too busy to take care of his tools.
>
> SPANISH PROVERB

16 *See your body as a valuable tool God has entrusted to your use.*

When I was young, I took my health for granted. Only when my body "let me down" for the first time did I understand how dependent I am on my body's strength and health.

Don't wait until your body is broken down before you pay attention to it. Keep it in good condition. Get enough sleep, eat nourishing food, and get regular exercise. Our bodies deserve at least as much regular maintenance as we give the tools we use for daily life—our cars, our kitchen utensils and appliances, our computers, whatever work tools we use—for we are far more dependent on this precious tool than on any other.

Study to shew thyself
approved unto God,
a workman that needeth
not to be ashamed.

2 TIMOTHY 2:15 KJV

17 *Think more about others.*

Sometimes we all lose our sense of perspective. We become so focused on ourselves and our flaws, we fail to see the needs in the world around us.

But when we stand in God's presence, I doubt His first concern is to have us jump on the bathroom scales. Instead, I suspect He's far more likely to ask, "What are you doing for others? How are you demonstrating My love?"

One thing I know:
The only ones among you who will be really happy
are those who will have sought
and found how to serve.

ALBERT SCHWEITZER

DIETING IN REAL LIFE

To make ourselves happy,
we must make others happy. . .
in order to become spiritually vigourous,
we must seek the spiritual good of others.
In watering others, we ourselves are watered.

CHARLES SPURGEON

Help us, O God, to do our best
to help other people to accomplish and achieve,
knowing that their contribution is what
God is trying to give the world.

FLORENCE SIMMS

> The sin of perfectionism is that it mutilates life by demanding the impossible.
>
> JEROME FRANK

18 *Give yourself credit for your accomplishments.*

I'm seldom satisfied with myself, particularly when it comes to my weight. No matter how much I achieve, I always know I have farther to go. If I lose that five pounds I was trying to drop, right away I turn my attention to the next five pounds I want to erase. No wonder I get exhausted with the entire process: I'm like a thirsting person staggering through the desert toward a mirage that constantly retreats.

In reality, each of my days is filled with tiny achievements. I need to recognize them, for little by little they will accumulate. But if I will accept only perfection and nothing less, I will always be discouraged. Inevitably, I will become frustrated. Eventually, I may give up altogether.

God doesn't want me to follow the mirage

of perfection. Instead, His grace gives me strength to walk forward step-by-step. And as I acknowledge each small step, I am refreshed.

Then God opened [Hagar's] eyes
and she saw a well of water.

GENESIS 21:19

Think of it—not one whorled finger
exactly like another! If God should take
such delight in designing fingertips,
think how much pleasure the unfurling
of your life must give Him.

LUCIE CHRISTOPHER

19 *Don't compare yourself to others.*

Each of us is unique—physically, emotionally,
intellectually. God is full of infinite, loving
creativity, and He never uses a cookie cutter
when He makes something (whether it's snow-
flakes or stars or human beings). He delights in
our idiosyncrasies.

So if God doesn't expect you to look or act
or be like anyone else, why should you expect
that of yourself?

DIETING IN REAL LIFE

God knew how much the world needed your smile,
Your hands, Your voice,
Your way of thinking,
Your insights, Your love.
God speaks through you in a way
He can through no other.
Be true to the person He created.

GWYNETH GAVIN

And God saw every thing that he had made,
and, behold, it was very good.

GENESIS 1:31 KJV

You are a part of the great plan,
an indispensable part.
You are needed; you have your own unique
share in the freedom of Creation.

MADELEINE L'ENGLE

> No great thing is created suddenly,
> any more than a bunch of grapes or a fig.
> If you tell me that you desire a fig,
> I answer that there must be time. Let it
> first blossom, then bear fruit, then ripen.
>
> EPICTETUS

20 Be patient with yourself.

I like immediate gratification; I'm easily discouraged when I have to wait for something. If the goal I have in mind doesn't materialize today. . .or next week. . .or even next year, I'm certain that means it will never materialize. So when it comes to losing weight, I've been quick to give up.

But if I look at the natural world, I see that immense results are often accomplished with immense slowness. Drop by drop and grain by grain, rock is shaped and canyons carved. Slowly, surely, the face of the earth is radically changed.

We, too, are being changed with the same slow sureness. We can afford to be patient with ourselves, for we are loved by a patient God. He

has all the time in the world to make us whole.
In fact, He has eternity.
    And so do we.

Have patience with all things,
but chiefly have patience with yourself.

Francis de Sales

Sometimes our fate resembles a fruit tree in winter.
Who would think at beholding such a sad sight
that those jagged twigs will turn green again
in the spring and blossom and bear fruit,
but we hope it, we know it.

Goethe

You grow up on the day you have
your first real laugh—at yourself.

ETHEL BARRYMORE

21 *Don't take yourself so seriously.*

The world will not end if you don't meet your
next diet goal. And life is filled with opportunities to laugh. It would be a shame if we were so
serious about our "diet journey" that we missed
all the funny things that happened along the way.

Take time to laugh.

Angels fly because
they take themselves lightly.

ANONYMOUS

> All changes, even the most longed for,
> have their melancholy, for what we
> leave behind us is part of ourselves.
> We must die to one life before
> we can enter another.
>
> ANATOLE FRANCE

22 *Trust God.*

For many of us, overeating has become a way of life. It may not be a healthy way to deal with life's stresses, but in some way, at some level, it has worked for us. It's helped us manage; it's how we've coped with life's ups and downs.

At the same time, we often hate this aspect of ourselves—and yet we're frightened to let go of it. How will we comfort ourselves when we are sad, how will we celebrate when we are happy, how will we stimulate ourselves when we are bored if we can't turn to food?

God holds the answers to those questions— but the answers may not be clear to us right now. We may even have to walk a long way in the dark before we find the light of understanding and knowledge.

But if we choose to trust God, then we can let go of this habit we've clung to so long. We can venture out into the dark. Sometimes that's the only way we can really find the light.

Fear clings. Faith lets go.

ELLYN SANNA, *Motherhood: A Spiritual Journey*

We glorify rugged wills;
but the greatest things are done
by timid people
who work with simple trust.

JOHN LA FARGE

CHAPTER 2
Changing Our Eating Habits

What is a diet? Something
you go on. . .to go off!

JANE BRODY

23 Don't diet, at least not in the traditional sense of the word.

Recent research indicates that miracle diet plans and quick-fix dieting solutions seldom do any lasting good. What's worse, drastic diets and diet pills that radically alter normal eating patterns may also disrupt brain chemicals. As a result, they may actually make your cravings worse.

If you gradually shift your eating habits a little at a time, you will "turn down" your body's appetite-control chemicals. Gradual weight loss also helps to burn body fat and keep off the weight.

You'll also be more successful if you avoid diets that tell you to eat only one or two foods to lose weight, as well as those that cut out entire food groups, such as fruits, vegetables, proteins, or carbohydrates. Stay away from diets that reduce your intake to less than 1,000 calories a day. Rigid diets that give you prescribed eating plans may help you lose weight—but eventually, you'll have to go back to your normal eating habits. That's when you'll probably find that the weight comes creeping back.

You need to *change your diet*, not *go on a diet*. This means creating new eating habits—and building habits takes time. Don't expect to do it all at once, in one drastic step. Such radical changes seldom last. Instead, make one or two adjustments in your eating habits each week.

> If you have formed the habit
> of checking on every new diet
> that comes along, you will find that,
> mercifully, they all blur together,
> leaving you with only one
> definite piece of information:
> French fried potatoes are out.
>
> JEAN KERR

Diet FACT

Researchers tell us that people who lose no more than one to two pounds a week are more likely to keep off the pounds.

24 *Learn to hear your body's messages.*

I need to eat. That's the message we hear after a long hard day. . .in the middle of a boring afternoon. . .when we're nervous. . .when we want to have fun with a friend. . .when we're sad. But what part of us is really sending that message to our consciousness?

We may assume it's our stomachs—but much of the time when we think we're hungry, it's not really our bodies that are talking to us. Instead, it's often our emotions (and they're actually asking for some other form of attention rather than food).

Most children and animals eat when they're hungry and stop eating when they're full. But as adults, many of us have grown deaf to our bodies' voices. We eat whether or not we're hungry, for other reasons besides our bodies' needs. And we keep eating even when our stomachs are full.

Listening to what your *body* wants is one of the first steps toward changing your diet. It may take some effort, for long ago most of us learned to tune out our bodies' messages while we listened instead to our emotions. At first, you will probably need to consciously ask yourself, *Am I really hungry? Am I full yet?* And then you will have to listen hard for the answers. Gradually, though, with practice, you will form new habits of thinking about food and hunger.

The good thing about this approach to eating is that it does not mean depriving yourself. Instead, it means giving your body what it *really* wants.

"My people will never again go hungry."

EZEKIEL 34:29 NLT

Another good reducing exercise consists
in placing both hands against the table edge
and pushing back.

ALEXANDER WOOLLCOTT

25 Only eat when you're hungry, and stop eating when you're full.

It sounds so obvious—and yet we all know it's so hard to practice, especially when we're offered one of our favorite foods. It may help if you tell yourself that today is not the last time that particular food will be available. Too often, we have a starvation mentality; we feel as though we have to eat as much as we can right now, as though this were our only chance to enjoy eating.

When I want to keep eating and eating at suppertime, I find I can stop myself more easily if I remind myself that I'll have more chances to enjoy eating tomorrow. As I look forward to my favorite breakfast or a lunch meeting with a friend, I can say no to the food I don't need right now. Besides, as Cervantes pointed out, food tastes better when we're hungry; when we eat for other reasons besides true hunger, the food we wanted so badly often cloys our tongues and sits like lead in our stomachs.

I think my greed for food also has a spiritual element. Remember when the Israelites could only gather the manna they needed for the day, rather than stockpiling it for the next day? By depending on God day by day, they learned to rely more on His providence and less on their own efforts—and I suspect we all need to do the same.

Our God longs to give us pleasure. We don't have to snatch and grab as much food as we can, like greedy children afraid there won't be enough to go around. Instead, as we learn to eat only what our bodies really need, we can grow in faith, relying on God to feed us tomorrow and the next day—physically, emotionally, spiritually—just as He has fed us today.

Saying *no thank you* is still
the best reducing exercise.

JOHN NEWTON BAKER

Then the LORD said...,
"I will rain down bread
from heaven for you."

EXODUS 16:4

Diet HINTS

After you've eaten your meal, get up from the table and clear the dishes. Don't allow yourself to continue nibbling on food you don't really need. The time to stop is just before you feel full.

If you are offered something to eat while you're a guest, but you're not *really* hungry, ask for a glass of ice water or a cup of tea instead. You don't need to offer any explanations; announcing that you are on a diet will only make both you and your host self-conscious.

26 *Eat more protein.*

A few years ago, I went on a high-protein, low-carbohydrate diet. Several friends were on the same diet, and we all had success; I lost eighteen pounds in about a month, and one woman in our group lost close to forty pounds in only a couple of months. We were all convinced that this was the way to diet—until we gradually returned to our regular eating habits and found that the weight crept back on. Eventually, we all tried to go back on that same high-protein diet—and found that this time around, we just couldn't do it. For emotional reasons, it seemed too extreme, too demanding—and we knew we didn't want to live like that forever. A few women even had physical reactions to the diet this time that meant they couldn't stick with the diet's requirements.

But I did benefit positively from this diet

experience: It taught me how little protein I eat normally and how much I was depending on carbohydrates to get me through the day. Left on my own, I was prone to eat starchy foods like bagels or muffins for breakfast and lunch and then have a single serving of protein for supper.

You may want to avoid extreme versions of diets. But that doesn't mean we can't learn something from these diets. As in all things, moderation is usually the best practice.

If you keep a food journal and find that you, too, are getting most of your daily calories from carbohydrates, you may want to consider increasing your protein intake. There are good reasons for doing so. After a protein-rich meal, the pancreas releases glucagon into the bloodstream. This chemical encourages your body to use its own reserves of stored fat for your energy requirements between meals. In other words, you're less likely to crave another quick-fix carbohydrate for energy—and you're more inclined to burn off the fat that's clinging to your thighs.

"You will know that it was the LORD
when he gives you meat to eat."

EXODUS 16:8

Diet FACTS

An average adult should consume per day at least 1 gram of protein for each 2.2 pounds (1 kilogram) of weight, somewhere between 55 and 70 grams (2 to 2.5 ounces) for the average woman.

All carbohydrates absorbed by the body are eventually converted to glucose—and glucose is the body's main fuel. It is either used immediately to provide energy or stored in the form of glycogen in the liver and in muscle to be utilized later. Any remaining glucose then is stored as fat.

When carbohydrates are broken down to glucose (sugar) in our body, our blood sugar goes up. Insulin is then secreted by the pancreas to lower our blood sugar; but in the process, insulin promotes the storage of fat and the elevation of cholesterol levels. Insulin also inhibits the loss of previously stored fat.

After you eat 50 to 100 grams of glucose during a high-sugar meal, your insulin levels will usually become very elevated and can remain so for several hours. Eating mostly high-carbohydrate meals can cause insulin to be elevated for most of the day—and this means your body is storing fat more often than using it.

> If the good Lord meant us
> to eat only sugar and honey,
> He'd have made us honey bees.
> We women have cheated ourselves for
> years—and now it's time we recognized
> that life holds plenty of sweetness.
> It's not only inside the sugar bowl
> (and the cookie jar)!
>
> LARENA WIGGINS

27 *Eat less refined sugar.*

Surprisingly, the percentage of fat consumed per person since the late 1970s has actually decreased from 40 percent to 33 percent—and yet the incidence of obesity has doubled since the late 1970s, and people weigh eleven to twelve pounds more than when they were consuming larger quantities of fat! Many researchers connect this trend to North Americans' sugar consumption.

Refined sugar did not exist anywhere in the world until around A.D. 500. In those long-ago times, an individual's pancreas gland was probably not called upon to secrete as much insulin in an entire lifetime as it is called upon in modern times to secrete nearly *every day!* Scientists tell us that most of our body fat comes from ingested sugar, not ingested fat.

I often turn to sugar as a quick fix for whatever ails my life. Sugar lifts my spirits. Because it changes my blood chemistry, I really do feel better—at least for awhile. All too soon, my emotions crash, leaving me with a headache and an uncomfortable stomach (not to mention the fat that accumulates around my waist and thighs).

I wonder what would happen if instead of eating something sweet, I took a few moments to go for a walk. . .put on my favorite music. . .hug my husband. . .or say a prayer.

Bad habits are trying to call
our attention to some
part of our lives that is
unlived or unexpressed.

SIDRA STONE

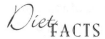

Diet FACTS

According to the U.S. Department of Agriculture, Americans consume approximately 150 pounds per person per year of refined sugar. (That is over one-third of a pound per person per day!)

The rate of diabetes in the United States has more than tripled since 1958. Recent statistics suggest that excess sugar consumption is either directly or indirectly causing diabetes.

I am the food of adults; grow,
and thou shalt feed upon Me.

AUGUSTINE

28 *Eat more complex carbohydrates.*

When you crave something sweet, try eating a complex carbohydrate instead. Researchers have found that when you eat a complex carbohydrate, it stimulates a greater loss of fat cells than when you eat the same amount of calories in another form. That means if you eat a plate of pasta, you'll actually be more likely to lose weight than if you ate the same amount of ice cream. A gram of carbohydrates has four calories compared to nine calories in a gram of fat, so it makes sense to fill up on complex carbohydrates rather than the same amount of fatty foods.

Complex carbohydrates can be as filling and satisfying as more fattening foods. And they are better for you.

Pay attention, my child, to what I say.
Listen carefully. Don't lose sight of my words. . .
for they bring life and radiant health.

PROVERBS 4:20–22 NLT

Diet FACTS

Carbohydrates come in two types: simple and complex, and both are built from units of sugar. You'll find simple carbohydrates in fruits, vegetables, milk, sugar, candy, and soft drinks. Complex carbohydrates are in grains (bread, cereal, rice, and pasta), starchy vegetables (potatoes, corn, and peas), and legumes (dried beans, peas, and lentils).

The Dietary Guidelines for Americans recommends six to eleven servings of complex carbohydrates a day, even when trying to lose weight. A serving size can be one slice of bread, one ounce of ready-to-eat cereal, or a half cup of pasta, rice, or cooked cereal.

29 Include dairy products in your diet.

Dairy products provide many of the vitamins necessary to good health. What's even better, though, is that experts now suggest that eating three servings of milk and dairy products a day can actually help prevent weight gain, and a diet rich in calcium can lead to weight loss over time.

Researchers recently analyzed the diets of thirty-two obese adults and found that those who ate three servings of dairy products a day lost 10.9 percent of their body weight, while those on calcium supplements lost only 8.1 percent, and those with little calcium or dairy in their diet lost a mere 6.4 percent, of their body weight. Overall, the adults who ate three servings of dairy products a day lost 64 percent more body fat (especially from their trunks or middle areas) than those who were dieting with no dairy products.

So drink your milk (and don't forget to nourish your soul with spiritual milk as well)!

Crave pure spiritual milk,
so that by it you may grow up in your salvation,
now that you have tasted that the Lord is good.

1 PETER 2:2–3

His fruit was sweet to my taste.

SONG OF SOLOMON 2:3

30 *Eat fruit.*

If you crave something sweet, try eating a piece of fruit instead of a cookie. Fruits are a great source of sugar because they generally don't stimulate insulin production as much as other sugars; what's more, they're not empty calories, because they also provide many of the vitamins we need for good health. Fruit is high in fiber, as well.

Keep lots of fresh fruit on hand. It makes a good snack to tide you over between meals, so you might want to put it in a bowl where you can see it. That way, you're more apt to reach for an apple or an orange—and less likely to stick your hand in the cookie jar.

This is what the Sovereign LORD showed me:
a basket of ripe fruit.

AMOS 8:1

Diet HINT

Many diet experts believe that fruits eaten by themselves are digested and absorbed at better rates than if eaten with other carbohydrates and fats. This means fruits will promote fat production less if you eat them as snacks rather than as part of a meal.

Diet FACT

The Dietary Guidelines for Americans recommends two to four servings of fruit each day. A serving equals:

1 medium banana, apple, or orange
(no bigger than a tennis ball)
½ cup of chopped, cooked, or canned fruit
¼ cup of dried fruit
¾ cup of fruit juice

Life consists not simply in what heredity
and environment do to us but in what we
make out of what they do to us.

HARRY EMERSON FOSDICK

> Fiber scours out your insides—it
> feels good between your teeth—
> and it satisfies the heart.
>
> JAMES JACOBS

31 *Eat more fiber.*

A bran muffin may have the same amount of calories as a doughnut—but the effect it has on your body may not be the same. By the same token, a bowl of oatmeal will be less apt to be converted to fat than two slices of white bread.

That's because foods containing insoluble fiber can affect your body's rate of digestion and absorption of carbohydrates. The fiber content keeps these carbohydrates from stimulating the production of insulin the way they would if they were eaten by themselves—and this in turn means that your body won't store as many of the calories as fat. This is obviously a good thing for your body.

Diet FACT

Recent research suggests that by doubling fiber intake from 12 to 24 grams a day (the USDA recommends 30 grams of fiber per day), an individual may burn an average of 90 more calories per day.

Diet HINT

Ways to include more fiber in your diet:

Read the labels of breakfast cereals carefully and go with those that have very little or no added sugar, the highest fiber or bran content, and the least processing of the grain.

When you eat pasta, use stone-ground whole-grain pasta.

If you crave crunchy snacks, try replacing potato chips with fiber-rich cereals mixed with a handful of tastier kids' sugarcoated cereals.

Add wheat germ and/or oat bran to home-made bread, meat loaf, even cookies and cakes.

> Fear the Lord and turn your back on evil.
> Then you will gain renewed health and vitality.
>
> PROVERBS 3:7–8 NLT

32 Eat less fat.

Some researchers suggest that merely by switching from a diet with 40 percent of total calories from fat to a diet with only 20 to 25 percent fat, an average, active person may steadily, permanently lose body fat without cutting back on overall calories.

This doesn't mean eat *no* fat, however. Surprisingly, fats, in and of themselves, do not necessarily cause weight gain. Moreover, fats are vitally important to our bodies, since they provide essential elements, such as fatty acids, many vitamins, and hormones important for metabolic processes. But researchers have found that most North Americans need to reduce their intake of saturated foods. Try to divide your fat "budget" evenly throughout the day.

Diet FACT

To calculate 25 percent of total daily calories in grams of fat per day, multiply your total daily calorie intake by 0.25 and divide the result by 9. For example, at 1,800 calories per day for a typical moderately active woman, total fat shouldn't exceed 50 grams.

Diet HINTS

If you eat creamy foods, you may not miss the fat. For instance, have a fruit-and-yogurt smoothie for a snack; eat a bowl of chowder for lunch. If you thicken soups with pureed potato, winter squash, or cornstarch and thicken a smoothie with a banana, these soups and smoothies can provide the creamy texture of fat and be filling without being fattening.

Choose fat-free or low-fat alternatives to traditional staples like sour cream, cream cheese, yogurt, cheese, peanut butter, luncheon meats, and whole wheat crackers. But beware! Carefully read labels on fat-free desserts; they are likely to be just as calorie-dense as original versions since they compensate for the fat by adding more sugar. Try not to fall into the mental trap of eating more than you would normally, justifying yourself with the fact that the food is low in fat.

Lettuce is like conversation:
it must be fresh and crisp....
You can put everything, and
the more things the better, into
salad as into a conversation.

CHARLES DUDLEY WARNER

33 Include salad and/or vegetables in every meal.

If you start your meal with a large helping of salad or vegetables, you'll fill yourself up with foods that are low in fats and calories and high in vitamins and fiber. That means you'll be less apt to overeat on other foods later in the meal—and you'll be sure to give your body what it needs before you give your appetite what it may think it wants.

Spinach is the broom of the stomach.

FRENCH PROVERB

Diet HINTS

Ways to include more vegetables in your diet:

Stir grated carrots, onions, mushrooms, and peppers into spaghetti sauce.

Add a layer of broccoli or spinach to lasagna in place of some of the meat or cheese layers.

Add green peas, carrots, celery, onion, bell peppers, squash, or sweet potatoes to casseroles.

Add carrots, tomatoes, or green beans to baked beans, chili, and meat loaf.

Add carrots, peas, peppers, or red onions to potato salad.

Add extra vegetables such as potatoes, corn, beans, peas, carrots, or squash to canned soups.

Stuff baked potatoes with spinach, broccoli, mushrooms, salsa, and low-fat yogurt.

Mix grated carrots, zucchini, corn, or green chilies into corn bread and muffin batter.

Skewer twice as many vegetables as extra-lean meat (chicken or shellfish) when making shish kebabs. Include mushrooms, carrots, eggplant, cherry tomatoes, zucchini, onion, and potato.

Try using a grilled Portobello mushroom marinated in olive oil, balsamic vinegar, minced garlic, and salt as an alternative to beef patties.

Rather than always steaming your vegetables, trying grilling or roasting them to accent their flavor and sweetness.

34 Eat "whole" foods.

Modern food processing includes puffing, intense mechanical treatments, and canning, all of which considerably alter the foods' fiber contents. Processing breaks down foods, making them more quickly absorbed by the body—and more easily converted into body fat.

Generally, foods that are less processed are less likely to be stored as body fat, since they don't encourage the production of insulin. Obviously, then, the more processing a carbohydrate such as rice, corn, or wheat has undergone, the more "fattening" will be its calories.

Think of whole grains and fresh fruits and vegetables as coming straight from God's hand, just as He intended them to be.

What I love most is
an abundance of simple food
of perfect quality and
staggering freshness,
very simply and respectfully treated,
tasting strongly of itself.

Sybille Bedford

> Happiness is essentially a state of going somewhere, wholeheartedly, one-directionally, without regret or reservation.
>
> WILLIAM H. SHELDON

35 Try to eat consistently from day to day.

All of us have times when we eat more than at other times (for instance, at family celebrations and holiday get-togethers). But if you make a habit of overeating one day and then compensate by undereating the next, you may actually slow down metabolism. Ultimately, this will make it that much harder to lose weight.

Imagine that at each meal you eat, Jesus is sitting down with you at the table. Whether you are alone or with others, be aware of His presence with you. You'll be less likely to either overeat or starve yourself when you realize Jesus is there at your side.

> I will be with you always.
>
> JESUS (MATTHEW 28:20)

36 *Don't count calories.*

Calories are not the answer to weight gain or loss. In 1980, a researcher named Webb tabulated a number of overeating studies and determined that energy intake (measured in calories) is not sufficient to predict weight gain or loss in any given individual. But our culture is still obsessed with calories. We love to measure things—and we forget that we sometimes lack the understanding to truly measure accurately.

Consuming and expending energy is a complex process. Researchers now know that decreasing the amount of calories in the diet only leads to temporary weight loss. In other words, eventually your body rebalances itself at its new level of caloric intake; otherwise, you would lose weight indefinitely by reducing calories—

and by the same token, by eating more calories, you would gain more and more weight until you weighed hundreds of pounds!

Eating healthy portions from all the food groups is a far more realistic way to achieve a healthy weight.

Don't let someone else dictate
the terms of your diet;
you need to find out how much
is right for you.

ANNE COLBY

Diet FACT

The term calorie was first used by Lavoisier in the 1840s. A calorie is the amount of energy (heat) needed to raise one kilogram of water one degree Centigrade (from 15°C to 16°C). In other words, it is a measure of the amount of energy required to achieve a certain result.

Diet **HINT**

If you need the concrete approach to dieting that counting calories provides, you might want to try instead a dieting tool like that offered by Weight Watchers®, where each food portion is assigned a point value that takes into account several factors (like fiber and fat content), rather than focusing only on calories.

> A person's palate can, in time,
> become accustomed to anything.
>
> NAPOLEON I

37 *Take your time as you change your eating habits.*

When I begin a diet, I'm apt to go from overeating one day to a strict food regimen the next. I feel very virtuous so long as I can stick to my new discipline—but as the days go by, it becomes harder and harder for me to conform to my diet plan. The cravings often become irresistible.

Dieting is not merely a matter of self-discipline. Like any addiction, our bodies (not to mention our emotions) may be dependent on getting their customary "fix." That's why we may need to gradually adjust our brain chemistry before we can hope to make any progress.

For instance, if you're accustomed to a large serving of something sweet late at night, going "cold turkey" may not be the answer, since your body will continue craving its regular dose of sugar. Instead, reduce the serving size and slowly substitute more nutritious foods for your bedtime snack. Your goal should be this: Eventually (not immediately), you either won't eat after dinner or you will choose only low-fat, low-sugar snacks.

Slow and steady wins the race.

AESOP

Diet HINTS

Eating salads is not necessarily a guarantee for weight loss if you pour on the salad dressing. If you drip one or two tablespoons of dressing (45 to 90 calories) onto your salad rather than pouring on four tablespoons (180 calories), think of all the calories you'll save. If you like your salad "wetter," use juicy tomatoes or add a little lemon juice. At restaurants, ask for your dressing on the side. At home, dilute creamy dressings with buttermilk and oil-based dressings with vinegar.

Rather than sautéing meat in oil, use defatted chicken broth, which adds wonderful flavor and cuts the fat content.

When roasting vegetables, place oil in a spray

bottle and mist the veggies rather than brushing on heavier amounts of oil.

When eating soups, stews, or chili, refrigerate them overnight and then skim the fat from the top the next day. Just one tablespoon of fat eliminates 115 calories and 13 grams of fat.

Use olive, sesame, or walnut oils in cooking, since they have a stronger flavor than other oils, allowing you to use less while not cutting taste.

To replace butter, make a spread out of roasted garlic cloves: Roast the top of a head of garlic sprinkled with water for 45 minutes at 350°. This will save you 68 calories or 8 grams of fat over what you would have consumed if you'd eaten two teaspoons of butter instead.

When baking muffins or quick breads, substitute applesauce for cooking oil. It creates moist and flavorful baked goods and saves you 152 calories or 18 grams of fat when compared to oil.

Use egg whites rather than whole eggs.

Substitute buttermilk for milk when baking.

Use half the nuts called for in a recipe.

Use ground turkey rather than ground beef to save 853 calories and 91 grams of fat per pound. (But be sure you use turkey *breast*. If your turkey includes dark meat and the skin, you will end up with more fat than lean ground beef.)

38 *Don't cut breakfast.*

Research reports that breakfast eaters tend to have less fat on their bodies—and what's more, they have greater energy and strength. Apparently, eating a healthy breakfast makes it easier to maintain a balanced diet—while skipping breakfast only increases your cravings later in the morning. By denying your body food until later in the day, you may also slow your metabolism; your body may go into starvation mode, holding on tight to excess body fat while it sends out desperate pleas for more high-fat foods. When you do eat, your body then stores fat, preparing for the next morning's famine.

Begin the day as you intend to continue.

LIZA DARIAN

Diet FACT

A recent study at Memorial University of Newfoundland suggests that eating breakfast also protects against morning heart attacks. According to this research, skipping breakfast increases platelet stickiness, which may promote clotting and contribute to heart attacks.

39 *Don't skip other meals, either.*

Your body needs fuel; it can't function at its best
if you deny it the calories it needs to work. And
surprisingly, eating multiple small meals actually helps your body let go of the fat it has
stored. Also, if you avoid getting desperately
hungry, you are less likely to binge when you
do eat.

Give thanks to the Lord of lords...
who gives food to every creature.
His love endures forever.

PSALM 136:3, 25

40 *Don't eat a large meal immediately before going to bed.*

Many diet experts believe that a large meal of any type should not be eaten just before going to bed. The calories you consume late in the day may be more likely to be stored as fat overnight, instead of being burned off through exercise. Instead, you should try to finish your evening meal by no later than 8:00 P.M. After that, consider the kitchen closed—no midnight snacks! You may also find you sleep better if your body isn't working on digesting its last meal while you are trying to rest.

In vain you rise early and stay up late, toiling for food to eat—for he grants sleep to those he loves.

PSALM 127:2

41 Eat smaller meals.

Sometimes the more we want, the less satisfied we are. It's a spiritual truth—and a diet fact, as well.

Large meals stimulate excessive insulin production—and insulin encourages your body to store fat. Moderate meals and even small between-meal snacks make your body handle calories in a more efficient and healthier way.

Better one handful with tranquillity than
two handfuls with toil
and chasing after the wind.

ECCLESIASTES 4:6

> A [woman] is rich in proportion
> to the things [she] can leave alone.
>
> HENRY THOREAU

42 Don't combine eating with other activities.

How many times do you eat while you drive. . .
read the paper. . .watch television. . .or work?
We're so busy that we often feel guilty simply
sitting down to enjoy our food, especially when
we're eating alone.

But when we don't allow ourselves to be fully
involved with eating, reveling in the conscious
pleasure to be found in each delicious bite of
food, we have a tendency to mindlessly take bite
after bite for twenty minutes. Eventually, our
stomachs will get through to our brains that we
are full. But if we're paying attention, we'll not
only take more pleasure in eating—we'll also
know when to quit.

DIETING IN REAL LIFE

We ask the blessing before we eat. . .
but we forget that God wants
to bless us while we eat.
We pack in enormous, unneeded quantities of food—
and all the while we miss the true savor
of what we are consuming.

Gwyneth Gavin

If the land floweth with milk and honey,
eat the honey and drink the milk, for both are thine.

Charles Spurgeon

> In general, mankind, since the improvement of cookery, eats twice as much as nature requires.
>
> BENJAMIN FRANKLIN

43 Read the labels on food packages.

Reading labels on processed or packaged foods is the only way you can tell what you're eating, especially since sugar is often added during processing or packaging. If an ingredient is not specifically listed in the grams column, you can sometimes estimate the amount, since ingredients are listed in order. For instance, if a sugar derivative, such as maltodextrin, is listed first or second, then you know that product has a high sugar content—which means it won't help you to lose weight.

> If we really knew what we were eating, we'd be less tempted to stuff our mouths with processed foods.
>
> CURT MICHAELS

Diet FACTS

Often, food labels claim that a product is fat free, low-fat, or light. Because these terms can be confusing, the Food and Drug Administration (FDA) has defined these terms:

Fat free: The product has less than 0.5 grams of fat per serving.

Low-fat: The product has 3 grams or less of fat per serving.

Reduced or *less fat:* The product has at least 25 percent less fat per serving than the full-fat version.

Lite or *light:* These terms can have a few meanings, so be careful. For instance:

The product has fewer calories or half the fat of the nonlight version.

The sodium content of a low-calorie, low-fat food is 50 percent less than the nonlight version.

A food is clearer in color (like light instead of dark corn syrup).

CHAPTER 3
Curbing Our Desires

> Knowledge is the first step to power.
>
> Janet Newman

44 Keep a journal of what you eat.

Researchers have found that people who write down everything they eat are more apt to change their eating habits on a long-term basis. They are the people who three years later have achieved and maintained their weight goals.

What about you? Have you ever eaten half a chocolate cake in one-inch pieces over the course of a day? Or have you found yourself sitting at the dinner table, devouring a second piece of lasagna straight from the serving dish, one forkful at a time?

I have. It's as though I think that if I break the food into small enough pieces, I'll cut out the calories. In my mind, I didn't have an entire piece of something—just a bite here and a bite there.

But if each time I take a bite of something, I record that in my food journal, then I avoid this rationalization. I'm also less inclined to do it in the first place, because it's just too much trouble writing down all those individual bites; for convenience's sake, I'm more apt to measure my food in reasonable portions.

Something about recording each bite of food we eat makes our eating more conscious. And if we can be more conscious of what we're doing, we often have more control of our actions.

> Once I write the truth in my journal,
> I find I can no longer use that particular
> rationalization for misbehavior.
> Once you know something,
> you can't unknow it.
>
> GWYNETH GAVIN

Diet FACT

A study published in the *New England Journal of Medicine* found that people who are overweight miscalculate their calories by an average of 47 percent.

> I groom myself in the bathroom;
> I sleep in the bedroom; I eat at the table.
> It makes life much more orderly.
>
> LIDA WILKES

45 Only eat when you're sitting down at the table.

Do you eat standing up at the kitchen counter while you do some other kitchen chore? Do you snack while you watch television? Do you nibble while you talk on the phone?

Try eating in only one or two specified places in your home. If you sit down at the table and focus on your food, rather than munching mindlessly anywhere and everywhere, you'll be more conscious of your food. You may even find you enjoy it more.

You prepare a table before me.

PSALM 23:5

> One should seek the company of only such people
> who call for the exercise of one's good behavior.
>
> ERNEST VON FEUCHTERSLEBEN

46

You may need to avoid the company of friends who encourage you to overeat, at least until your new habits are firmly established.

Do you have friends who insist you have a brownie to go with your coffee whenever you meet? Or does your time together always consist of munching on potato chips and dip? When you visit their home, do they press food on you until you accept?

Hospitality and food are firmly connected in many people's minds. These are the people who would never think of entertaining friends without encouraging them to eat. Still other friends may feel threatened by your new attitudes toward food; their own guilt will be alleviated if you break down and indulge with them.

You can explain to your friends that you are trying to learn different eating habits. But be prepared for the fact that they may not understand or accept your new way of living. Be ready to stand up for what is best for you— even if that means avoiding their company (as tactfully as possible) until your own resolve is less shaky.

My son, if sinners entice you,
do not give in to them.

PROVERBS 1:10

> Don't let your desires cloud your judgment.
>
> LANCE TIERRA

47 Learn to accurately judge the size of your portions.

Learn how to translate portion sizes from ounces or tablespoons into everyday objects you can mentally picture. And don't rely on restaurant-size portions for your concept of how much you're eating. Restaurant servings have swelled over the last few years, so be aware that a 32-ounce soft drink is actually equivalent to four normal servings; oversized muffins and bagels are actually two portions of carbohydrates, not one.

Many diet experts believe that using appropriate portions at each meal is more important (and more effective) than counting calories. The portions of food that you select for each meal should fit comfortably on a normal dinner plate, with nothing overlapping the sides. Once you have served your plate so that you have a meat, a vegetable, and a carbohydrate, all nicely arranged on your plate, do not go back for seconds or thirds.

Diet FACT

By choosing a 3-ounce steak instead of a 6-ounce steak, you can cut 225 calories; going with an 8-ounce glass of soda rather than a 32-ounce glass can reduce caloric intake by 500 calories.

Diet HINT

Use your hand to help you determine portion sizes:

Your palm (without the fingers) is roughly equal to a 3-ounce portion of meat, fish, or poultry.

Your fist equals 1 cup or one fruit.

A single handful equals 1 to 2 ounces of nuts or pretzels.

Your thumb is about the size of 1 ounce of meat or cheese.

48

*Avoid eating very little during
the day, only to stuff
yourself at night.*

During the day when I'm busy, it's easy for me
to eat lightly or even skip meals. As I breeze
out the door with only a cup of coffee, I often
feel quite virtuous about foregoing a more sub-
stantial (and nutritious) meal. On my most
hectic days, a diet soda and a piece of fruit
keep me satisfied at lunchtime—and again, I
think smugly about all the calories I'm cutting.

But by the end of that busy day, I'm ravenous. I'm exhausted and longing for a chance to
relax and have fun—and after eating so little
all day, I feel justified in consuming an enormous meal.

You can imagine my disappointment when I discovered that one of those immense meals I was eating often held nearly double the calories I'd have eaten had I enjoyed three normal meals spaced throughout the day!

What lies in our power to do,
it lies in our power not to do.

ARISTOTLE

> And it is well to eat slowly:
> The food seems to be more plentiful,
> probably because it lasts longer.
>
> M. F. K. FISHER

49 *Eat slowly, savoring every bite.*

We North Americans often think that quantity is better than quality. That may be why we feel cheated by small meals, no matter how delicious they may be. We eat quickly, our minds on other things, and we eat a lot.

But if you eat slowly, you have time to really enjoy your food—and you're less likely to feel as though you are depriving yourself by limiting your portion sizes. What's more, you will have more time to hear what your body is really telling you. It takes awhile for the message to get from your stomach to your brain that you've eaten enough—and if you are eating fast, you may have already eaten more than you really want by the time you realize your stomach is full.

The strong [woman] is the one
who is able to intercept at will the communication
between the senses and the mind.

NAPOLEON BONAPARTE

Diet FACT

A recent study by Theresa Spiegel, Ph.D., at the University of Pennsylvania, reported that people who increased the length of their meal by an average of about four minutes lost more body fat than those who ate more quickly.

Now the Lord will feed them
as a lamb in a large place.

HOSEA 4:16 KJV

Diet HINT

Before the main course of your meal, drink a glass of water or iced tea, eat a salad with low-fat dressing, or have a bowl of soup. If you fill a portion of your stomach with these no-calorie or low-calorie substances, you'll take the edge off your hunger. And you'll be less apt to overeat once you get to the more fattening food.

The uneasiness of hunger
can be more quickly removed
by a bowl of good soup than by any
other variety of food.

J. B. AND L. E. LYMAN

> Things forbidden have a secret charm.
>
> Tacitus

50 Treat yourself occasionally to small pieces of chocolate.

A Hershey Kiss or ten chocolate chips contain a surprisingly small amount of fat and calories—and they may help you fight off your cravings for a high-sugar, high-fat binge. Allowing yourself one small treat each day is important psychologically, since it helps you feel less deprived and frustrated.

But be careful. Don't put the open bag of chocolates within easy reach while you work, telling yourself that you'll only eat one or two. Like an alcoholic who can't stop after the first drink, you're likely to find that before you know it, you've eaten half the bag.

Instead, carefully take out only the small portion you're allowed and put the rest away. I find the bottom of our chest freezer is a good place for me to keep chocolate chips—or you might want to try the top shelf of a cupboard, someplace high enough where you can't reach it without standing on a step stool. The harder it is for you to get to it, the less likely you will be to yield to temptation.

Make that moment of small indulgence a tiny ceremony, one that you anticipate ahead of time. Stop everything you are doing and really pay attention to the delicious taste of chocolate on your tongue. Then go back to whatever your day holds, knowing that tomorrow—and the next day, and the day after that—you will be allowed that same moment of pleasure all over again.

And he shall stand and feed
in the strength of the LORD.

MICAH 5:4 KJV

> "But I will bring Israel back to his own pasture
> and. . .his appetite will be satisfied."
>
> JEREMIAH 50:19

51 Remove cues that make you feel like eating (such as treats and snacks lying about in dishes and bowls).

Empty the candy dishes. Put away the cookie jar. Don't leave bags of chips on the kitchen counter.

Instead, make an effort to fill your home with healthy cues for eating. Put a fruit bowl on the table. Keep a container of raw veggies on your desk while you work. Make sure that your food and your home are arranged in such a way that it's easier for you to pick up low-fat, nutritious foods—and more difficult to get your hands on sweet, fattening snacks.

52 *Drink plenty of water.*

Diet experts have found that drinking generous amounts of water is the number-one way to reduce food cravings and control appetite. Although recent research indicates that we don't really need those eight glasses a day that we heard so much about for years, it is still important to keep your system well-watered.

Our bodies sometimes confuse thirst with hunger. What you interpret as a craving for sweets may actually be a signal that your body needs fluids. Some people have even found that their cravings for ice cream subside after they drink one to two glasses of cold water.

"The LORD will guide you always....
You will be like a well-watered garden."

ISAIAH 58:11

Diet TIP

Drinking a glass of water may seem boring—
but you can make your water a treat by adding
lemon, lime, or orange slices, or by using ice
cubes that have been frozen with strawberries
or cherries in the center.

Jesus saith unto them,
Come and dine.

JOHN 21:12

53

*Use alternative flavorings—
like vanilla, nutmeg, spearmint,
cinnamon, and anise—
instead of sugar.*

Our tongues have been trained to consider bland food boring. But instead of automatically reaching for the sugar bowl the next time you have a bowl of oatmeal, try a few drops of vanilla instead. When you bake, experiment with reducing the amount of sugar and increasing the spices. Try adding a sprinkle of cinnamon or nutmeg to your coffee instead of sugar. Gradually, you'll develop new tastes—and you'll curb your craving for sweet foods.

Diet TIP

Tasty spices and how to use them:

Allspice: seasons muffins, breads, carrots, winter squash, and sweet potatoes.

Anise: provides licorice flavor to breads and desserts.

Cardamom: used in curries, winter squash, sweet potatoes, breads, cakes, cookies.

Cinnamon: adds spicy flavor to hot beverages, used in baked goods, fruit sauces, stews, puddings, carrots, sweet potatoes, and baked apples.

Cloves: flavors beverages, beets, carrots, sweet potatoes, winter squash, baked goods, meats, stews, and soups.

Coriander (or cilantro): good in salads, casseroles, soups, and stews.

Ginger: adds spice to marinades, steamed vegetables, chicken, or fish.

Mace: similar to nutmeg only milder (it's the fibrous covering on the nutmeg seed), enhances the flavor of broccoli, carrots, and cauliflower, brussels sprouts, baked goods, and puddings.

Nutmeg: brings out the flavor in spinach, broccoli, cauliflower, carrots, brussels sprouts, sweet potatoes, sauces, pasta, and stews.

> Don't be afraid to
> color outside the lines.
> Experiment. Be creative.
> Leave the old ways behind.
> Only then will you find
> the new roads that
> lead to health.
>
> LYDIA MAKEPEACE

54 *Experiment with ways to add flavor to your meals without adding calories.*

Here are some suggestions:

Add canned chilies to soups, sandwiches, or scrambled eggs.

Add canned roasted peppers to sandwiches or blend with cayenne and use as topping with cheese for crackers.

Use fresh cilantro in salsa, soups, dressings, and salads.

Use sun-dried tomatoes in pasta salads, sandwich spreads, and vegetable dips.

Use fresh ginger with curry to flavor chicken, or add to tea, stir-fry dishes, or salad dressings.

Mix balsamic vinegar with soups, pasta salads, or salad dressings.

Use horseradish in potato dishes, dips, soups, or on turkey burgers.

Use lemon zest to marinate fish, or add to sorbets, yogurts, and fruit salads.

Fresh dill, oregano, basil, and rosemary are delicious flavorings for pasta, vegetables, fish, and meat.

Mix apricot preserves into fruit salads or roll into a crepe with sour cream.

Use hazelnut or walnut oils instead of olive oil in vinaigrettes, in potato salad instead of mayonnaise, and on steamed vegetables.

Toss fresh mint with new potatoes, peas, or steamed carrots. Use mint to flavor iced tea or fresh fruit.

Drizzle honey over fruit salads, or use with olive oil, vinegar, and mustard for a vinaigrette.

55 Identify your trigger foods.

What foods are the hardest for you to resist? For me, it's hot fudge sundaes and pizza. So if I'm having lunch with a friend, I'm less apt to over-indulge if we meet at a place that serves hearty soups and salads than if we meet at our favorite pizza joint or the restaurant that offers ice cream at the end of every meal.

Don't rely on your willpower alone. Often seeing something—or smelling it—is enough to fuel our cravings. Avoid the temptation by steering clear of the dessert tray or the dough-nut shop. Plan ahead when you anticipate situations you know will tempt you. You'll be more successful at changing your diet if you can avoid the temptation altogether.

And lead us not into temptation.

MATTHEW 6:13 KJV

133

56 Don't go grocery shopping on an empty stomach.

If you grocery shop when you're ravenous, you'll have a harder time resisting all the foods that tempt you most. But if you shop when your stomach is full and satisfied, you'll make your selections using your intellect rather than your cravings. By exercising self-control in the grocery store, you'll be sure that in your weaker moments, the choices available to you are limited to healthy alternatives.

Make a practice of keeping tempting foods out of your house. If you know you can't resist it, don't buy it.

Perseverance must finish its work
so that you may be mature and complete

JAMES 1:4

To lengthen thy life, lessen thy meals.

BENJAMIN FRANKLIN

57 Keep your hunger from becoming overwhelming by eating small meals and snacks evenly distributed throughout the day.

You're less likely to overeat if you don't let yourself get too hungry. Plan your day around several small meals, with healthy snacks spaced between. This keeps on an even keel the chemicals in your body that send hunger messages.

What one has to do usually can be done.

ELEANOR ROOSEVELT

The wilderness yieldeth food
for them and for their children.

JOB 24:5 KJV

58 *Think before you eat.*

Don't try to ignore your hunger. Instead, pay attention to it—but never satisfy it mindlessly. Whenever you feel your body demanding food, ask yourself what specific food would satisfy your craving. What is it you really want? (Something crunchy? Something sweet? Something cold? Something salty?) Then determine a healthy way to give your body what it wants and eat a moderate-sized portion of that food.

Knowledge is power.

FRANCIS BACON

> Going slowly does not stop one from arriving.
>
> FULFULDE PROVERB

59 *Whenever your mind begins to obsess on fattening foods, focus your attention on your goal.*

Sometimes when I'm dieting, all I can think about is food. I wake up thinking about food; I go to sleep thinking about food. I think about food while I work; thoughts of food even intrude while I'm praying.

When this happens, I find it helps to replace the thoughts of food that haunt my mind with images of a thinner, healthier me. It's good to remind myself of just what my goal really is—and that obsessing on food is counterproductive to that goal. (I'll never achieve that more fit version of myself if I continue to behave as though consuming the largest number of brownies possible were my only goal!)

Goals are important. They keep us motivated;

they keep us heading in the right direction. But it's also important not to set your goals too high. Set yourself mini goals, things you can easily achieve *today*. If losing fifty pounds is your only objective, you're likely to become discouraged and frustrated (and possibly turn to food for comfort).

Even the most disciplined people have a limited capacity for self-control. Don't set yourself up for failure. Instead, give yourself small, easy-to-achieve daily and weekly goals, things you can realistically accomplish. These small milestones (like eating half a cup of ice cream instead of three scoops—or half a brownie instead of two whole ones) will eventually create the healthier person you hope to achieve.

You have to have a goal or you're not going anywhere.

BONNIE BLAIR

You can only see one thing clearly, and that is your goal.
Form a mental vision of that and cling to it
through thick and thin.

KATHLEEN NORRIS

Feed me with food
convenient for me:
Lest I be full, and
deny thee, and say,
Who is the LORD?

PROVERBS 30:8–9 KJV

60 *Pray before you eat.*

In a religious community, bells call people to prayer. In psychological terms, the ringing bell is the stimulus that triggers the prayer response.

Learn to think of hunger as your personal prayer bell. When you feel like eating, immediately turn your heart to God. Instead of thinking of hunger as a temptation, consider it a spiritual cue.

And when your heart is focused on God, He can help you determine what your body and emotions really need—whether it's physical, spiritual, or emotional food.

"He provides you with plenty of food
and fills your hearts with joy."

ACTS 14:17

He that has energy to root out a vice should go further,
and try to plant a virtue in its place.

CHARLES CALEB COLTON

Diet HINT

Chew sugarless gum while cooking or when you know you're going to be tempted to nibble. You'll be less tempted to mindlessly graze on fattening foods if you already have something in your mouth!

When patterns are broken, new worlds emerge.

TULI KUPFERBERG

> It is not immoral not to finish a meal,
> but it is of questionable morality
> to treat yourself like a
> waste-disposal system.
>
> JANE BRODY

61 *Don't clean your plate.*

I was raised to always eat everything on my plate. My parents were children of the Great Depression, and they would never have dreamed of "wasting" food.

But if we eat when we are no longer hungry, then we are actually wasting food, for it will only be used to store unnecessary fat. We need to learn to stop eating when we are comfortably full—even if there is still food on our plates.

> Progress is impossible without change.
>
> GEORGE BERNARD SHAW

62 *Never socialize on an empty stomach.*

We all tend to eat more when we're with friends and family. So if you're going to a family gathering or a get-together with friends, have a healthy snack before you leave. If you're not ravenous when you arrive, you'll find it easier to resist your mother's cooking and your friend's appetizers. (You might also want to avoid alcohol when you're socializing, since even one drink can undermine the best of intentions, leaving you more likely to overeat.)

63 *Get enough rest.*

When I'm overwhelmed by the number of things that have to be done in my day, I frequently cut out the moments where I would normally rest. *I don't have time for that,* I tell myself. I stay up late and get up early, trying desperately to cram more moments into my day. As a result, I'm exhausted. My tired body craves energy.

Those are the days when a little voice whispers inside my head: *Go ahead, have some Oreos. Eat some ice cream. Have a doughnut with your coffee. You deserve it after working so hard. You* need *it.*

But what my body really needs isn't a lot of empty calories. It needs rest. And when I stop shortchanging it of the rest it needs, I find that my cravings for high-sugar, high-fat foods diminish.

What's important is finding out
what works for you.

HENRY MOORE

64

The next time you're tempted to binge, imagine that someone you respect is watching you.

I'm much more apt to eat six brownies when I'm by myself than if I'm eating with my husband. And if I catch his eye as I'm reaching for yet another slice of pizza, I find myself suddenly able to restrain myself. It's not that I'm afraid of what he'll say; I'm just embarrassed to have him see me eating in ways that aren't healthy. Unfortunately, he's not with me all the time. And when the cat's away. . . But I've found that if I imagine someone sees me as I'm ripping open the chocolate chip bag, I'm less likely to find myself eating a quarter of the bag while I make chocolate chip cookies.

Imaginary people are easy to ignore, of course. But then I remind myself: Imagination may make God's presence seem more real to me—but He is my friend who is truly always with me, always watching.

And when I'm truly aware of God's holiness surrounding me, why would I want to cram chocolate chips in my mouth anyway?

We will glory in the presence
of our Lord Jesus.

I THESSALONIANS 2:19

CHAPTER 4
Spending More Calories

When we do the best that we can,
we never know what miracle
is wrought in our life.

HELEN KELLER

65 Make exercise a priority in your life.

When our lives are busy (which they often are), all too often exercise is the first thing we drop. We just don't have time to get up that extra hour or half hour earlier. . .we're just so tired after work. . . . The excuses are all too familiar. We may think we could make exercise a priority if only circumstances would cooperate—but the truth is, we make time for the things that are really our priorities.

Priorities are those basic, take-them-for-granted actions that we wouldn't dream of skipping. For instance, most of us demonstrate our commitment to cleanliness, because no matter how busy our lives, we still take the time to shower regularly. Hopefully, we also show our families they are priorities by never being too busy to kiss our husbands or hug our children.

I wouldn't dream of not brushing my teeth and putting on my makeup in the morning. I also find time to clothe myself appropriately, and I rarely miss my morning cup of coffee. If I can make time for those activities, then I can also squeeze at least a twenty-minute exercise session into even the busiest days.

Exercise is. . .about. . .honoring the
really important priorities in your life.
Your family and friends are the genuine treasures in life.
You, in turn, are their greatest gift.
Take care of your gift to them by acknowledging
that your body needs care and attention.

PAMELA PEEKE

Exercise FACT

In order to lose five pounds in one month, your body must register a loss of about 570 calories per day—and 570 calories is equivalent to a large order of French fries—or the amount you would burn if you spent an hour cross-country skiing each day.

Habit is habit, and not to be flung out
of the window by any [woman], but
coaxed downstairs a step at a time.

66 Begin slowly.

Don't start by trying to change your exercise
habits drastically, all at once. Instead, take small
steps toward a new commitment to exercise.

[She] who wants to do everything
will never do anything.

ANDRÉ MAUROIS

Exercise is not about trudging to your workout,
getting sore muscles, rushing around the gym.
It's about moving your body every day.

PAMELA PEEKE

67 Have realistic exercise expectations for yourself.

Highly structured routines may overwhelm you—and they may also be impossible to maintain. Don't set yourself up for failure by placing your expectations too high. Elaborate, rigid exercise plans are not as effective as stealing a few minutes here and there wherever possible to simply take a walk or ride your bike. Keep your goals manageable.

Small opportunities are often
the beginning of great enterprises.

DEMOSTHENES

Exercise HINT

Ways to work exercise into your daily life:

Instead of looking for the parking space nearest to the store, seek out the one that's the farthest away.

Use the stairs instead of the elevator.

Run up and down stairs as often as you can during the day.

When you have to run errands, walk to as many as you can and leave your car behind.

Combine exercise and household chores by vacuuming, mowing the lawn, or mopping the floor.

Perform without fail what you resolve.

BENJAMIN FRANKLIN

68 Do some form of aerobic exercise for at least 20 minutes four times a week.

Researchers have discovered that regular aerobic exercise, the kind that increases your heart and respiration rates, also helps you burn fat more quickly. What's more, you'll find that it increases your energy levels and reduces your stress. It also helps you build strength and bone density.

Exercise FACT

Aerobic exercise lowers insulin levels, as well as improving our cardiovascular systems. For maximum benefits, you should elevate your resting heart rate to a prescribed level for a period of twenty consecutive minutes. To determine your ideal heart rate during exercise, subtract your age from 220 and multiply this number by 0.70.

> [She] is my friend who succoreth me,
> not [she] that pitieth me.
>
> THOMAS FULLER

69 *Exercise with friends.*

Friends can help motivate you to stick with an exercise program. Instead of always meeting friends over a meal, get together for exercise. Go for a hike in the woods or a long walk through the neighborhood and talk along the way; ride bikes together; join a fitness club together. If exercise is a regular "date," you'll be less tempted to skip your exercise session.

> The best breakfast is a breath of
> morning air and a long walk.
>
> HENRY DAVID THOREAU

70 *Choose a convenient exercise activity that involves little equipment and expertise—like walking.*

The more complicated you make your exercise program, the more apt you will be to postpone practicing it. You may spend days and even weeks shopping for just the right equipment, daydreaming about the "new you"—but in the meantime you're missing the best opportunity to get moving: right now.

No matter where you are, you can walk. You can walk on city streets and country roads, the length of shopping malls and along quiet paths in the park. It really doesn't matter where you walk, so long as you're using your muscles regularly to move. Use your walking time to think. . .plan. . .pray.

71 *Lift weights.*

According to researchers, if you lift weights for 25 minutes three times a week, you will lose two pounds of fat and add one pound of muscle. This means you may weigh the same, but since muscle takes up less space than fat, you'll actually look thinner.

Lifting weights also increases your resting metabolic rate—the speed at which you burn off calories. After three months of weight lifting, this rate will go up by 7 percent, which means you will continue to lose fat.

Exercise HINT

A good rule of thumb in determining the appropriate weight for you to be lifting: Your muscles should feel tired after 15 repetitions.

72 Exercise when you get the urge to eat.

Most of us who struggle with our weight experience intense food cravings. Whenever the urge to eat hits you, try exercising instead. People who exercise regularly maintain a more constant weight and are less prone to binge eating. Exercise can also lift your spirits just as much as the richest dessert—and it's a far healthier alternative for reducing stress.

To remain young one must change.

ALEXANDER CHASE

Each day is a new life.
Seize it. Live it.

DAVID GUY POWERS

73 Exercise for at least five minutes after breakfast.

According to exercise experts, even a short burst of exercise can turn on your body's "thermic switch." In other words, exercise speeds up your metabolism. Some dietitians theorize that your body's metabolism slows down while you sleep—but exercise gets it going again, so that you'll burn more calories throughout your day.

Don't worry if you broke all your good resolutions yesterday. Each morning is a chance to start all over again.

Each day the world is born anew for him
who takes it rightly.

J. B. PRIESTLY

Each day is a little life;
every waking and rising a little birth;
every fresh morning a little youth.

ARTHUR SCHOPENHAUER

> It is common sense to take a method and try it.
> If it fails, admit it frankly and try another.
> But above all, try something.
>
> FRANKLIN D. ROOSEVELT

74 Take time to figure out the exercise program that's best for you.

Different forms of exercise appeal to different people. For instance, I like to take long walks, and I've never been much good at sports. My sister-in-law, on the other hand, is bored by walking, and she loves to play softball and basketball. If I had to join a softball league, I'd dread the games as much as my sister-in-law would dread having to walk. But I look forward to my daily walk—and my sister-in-law looks forward to meeting with friends to shoot hoops.

You, too, need to find a form of exercise that will be fun rather than a chore. If you've let all physical activity drop from your life, finding something that's right for you may take some experimentation—but eventually, you want to find something that will fit into your life permanently.

What's a joy to the one is a nightmare to the other.

BERTOLT BRECHT

Why not be oneself? . . . If one is a greyhound, why try to look like a Pekingese?

EDITH SITWELL

Exercise FACT

Finding the right exercise is more than just a matter of taste. What works for one person physically may not produce the same results for you; factors such as age, diet, fitness level, exercise intensity, hormonal changes, and gender play a part in the success of your efforts. Ask your doctor for her advice before beginning.

Habit is stronger than reason.

GEORGE SANTAYANA

75 *Create exercise habits.*

If you can stick with an exercise program for three or four weeks, you will have established a new habit—and once you have a new routine, willpower becomes less important.

Habits aren't formed overnight, so be patient with yourself. Persevere—and eventually, the power of habit will keep you going.

You didn't achieve your career goals
or raise your children overnight;
you are not going to become physically fit
overnight. . . . Women often expect to change
overnight, and the media has led them to
believe this transformation is quick and easy.
But. . .nothing meaningful or sustainable
is accomplished with shortcuts and quick fixes.

PAMELA PEEKE

76 Use vacations as a chance to exercise more rather than less.

I've established a healthy routine for my work-
days that includes healthy eating and regular
exercise—but unfortunately, any change in my
regular routine also disrupts my healthier
lifestyle. Vacations are particularly difficult. I
eat too much—and I exercise haphazardly. I
seem to look on vacations as a time to escape
healthy practices as well as my work.

That doesn't make much sense. Vacations
are meant to be times of refreshment and
renewal—but if we overeat and don't exercise
while we're on vacation, we're prone to come
home feeling heavy and tired.

Instead, exercise should be a fun part of our
vacation. It may take a little forethought—but we
can do it. We can skip the tour buses and do our
sightseeing on foot. Instead of lazing all day on the

beach, we can go for long walks beside the ocean. We can tour museums and historic churches. We can swim, play tennis, go skiing. . . .

And if we build exercise into our vacation, at the end of the day, we can enjoy a special meal without guilt.

Exercise FACT

When you get several good workouts each week, you can afford to eat a little more. Not only are you burning off calories and fat while you exercise, but you are speeding up your metabolism. So seize every opportunity for exercise that you can.

> Dear friend, I am praying that
> all is well with you and that your
> body is as healthy as I know your soul is.
>
> 3 JOHN 2 NLT

77

*Try to move around for at least
five minutes after every meal.*

Participating in an aerobics class, swimming, or running three miles a few times each week—or even once every day—is good for your health; but according to some exercise experts, it may not be the most effective way to boost your metabolism twenty-four hours a day. The period of intense activity will increase your metabolism briefly, but if you act as though you have "finished" with exercise until the next time, your resting metabolism is likely to return to its previous low level. When, instead, you walk briskly for five minutes after eating each meal, you may double the number of calories you burn for the next three hours or more.

> Dare to begin!
> [She] who postpones living rightly
> is like the rustic who waits for the river
> to run out before [she] crosses.
>
> HORACE

78

Have a Plan B in place for when your regular exercise plan is disrupted.

My life's been pretty disrupted lately. Health crises in my extended family have kept me traveling back and forth across the state; a business trip looms on the future's horizon; and physically, I haven't been feeling all that great myself. I'm tired and stressed, and exercise seems to require more self-discipline than I have right now. When life gets back to normal, I tell myself, then I'll begin exercising again.

Unfortunately, our lives are seldom "normal." In fact, we should learn to consider chaos and disruptions to be the normal state of affairs.

That being the case, we need to continue to make exercise a priority even when our normal routines are shattered.

This may mean using a hotel exercise room. It may mean walking around and around the same city block—or even running up and down flights of hospital stairs. When we're facing a personal or professional crisis, exercise may seem like the last thing on our list of priorities—but exercise will help us cope better, both physically and emotionally, with the demands of our circumstances.

If you will. . .remember that every experience
develops some latent force within you,
you will grow vigorous and happy,
however adverse your circumstances
may seem to be.

JOHN R. MILLER

> Victories that are cheap are cheap.
> Those only are worth having which
> come as the result of hard fighting.
>
> HENRY WARD BEECHER

79 *Be willing to pay the price for being physically fit.*

Our culture tries to make things convenient. We like things as easy as possible, as fast as possible. New and improved laborsaving appliances are constantly being produced; our computers work faster and faster; and even our food comes in an assortment of "instant" varieties.

But building a fit body is not a fast or easy endeavor. There are no shortcuts, no overnight solutions. If you want to look and feel different, there's a price to be paid. When you are willing to pay only a very little in terms of time and effort, then your results will also be meager.

Are you willing to pay the price?

Women who can routinely
find the baseline amount of time
to care for their bodies feel and appear
more energetic, vibrant, and centered,
and they look fit and terrific!
Pay the price and reap the rewards.

PAMELA PEEKE

> I must govern the clock,
> not be governed by it.
>
> GOLDA MEIR

80 Find the time of day that's best for you to exercise.

Are you a morning person? Or are you the sort of person who can barely function until after ten o'clock in the morning? What about your schedule? Are your mornings busier than your evenings?

Establishing an exercise program is hard enough without making it more challenging than it needs to be. Determine the time of day when it will work best for you. Try to match your exercise sessions to the times when you have the most energy. If you have schedule conflicts, see if there's any way you can rearrange your responsibilities. You will probably need your family members' cooperation—but that's okay. You do plenty for them—it's all right for you to ask their help with this.

81 *Make exercise appointments with yourself.*

Sometimes, it seems impossible to fit everything into our busy days. Most time management experts recommend that you keep a daily planner as a tool for ensuring that at least the most important tasks are accomplished each day.

When you sit down with your planner and map out the week ahead, you need to write in your exercise times. If you don't plan ahead, they'll rarely happen.

82 Keep an exercise journal.

Include in your journal these factors:

How long you exercised.
What form your exercise took.
What time of day you exercised.
How you felt before you exercised.
How you felt during your exercise.
How you felt after.

A journal will give you feedback on how
your exercise plan is shaping up. You will be
able to see what works best—and what doesn't.
And a concrete record of your past achievement
will encourage you to keep going.

Exercise HINT

Combine your exercise journal with your food journal to give you an accurate overall picture of your journey toward a healthier lifestyle.

You will never "find" time for anything.
If you want time you must make it.

CHARLES BUXTON

Learn to use ten minutes intelligently.
It will pay you huge dividends.

WILLIAM A. IRWIN

83 Stretch.

If you break up your day with simple stretches (when you first get up, once or twice during your workday, and before you go to bed), you will build flexibility, balance, and strength—which will help your more vigorous exercise sessions go more easily. Stretching also reduces stress, so you may not be as tempted to reach for a candy bar or a cookie.

The real secret of how to use time
is to pack it as you would a suitcase,
filling up the small spaces with small things.

SIR HENRY HADDOW

> This above all: to thine own self be true.
>
> WILLIAM SHAKESPEARE

84 *Think of exercise as something positive you do for yourself; don't exercise out of guilt.*

Guilt is a cruel taskmaster. It will only motivate us for so long, because eventually, inevitably, we become resentful and rebellious. Inside us all lurks a cross child that's tired of having to obey all the rules.

So don't make your exercise routine one more rule you have to follow in order to appease that cruel taskmaster. Instead, think of it as one of the best gifts you could give yourself. Exercise not because you *ought* to—but because you're worth it!

> If I trim myself to suit others,
> I will soon whittle myself away.
>
> ANONYMOUS

CHAPTER 5
Dieting and Our Emotions

85 *Be aware that your emotions are linked to your diet.*

We often eat because we're depressed. When we do, we create a vicious circle: Our poor eating habits can lead to mood swings, poor concentration, and fatigue, which in turn result in more poor food choices.

Don't wait until you feel happier to begin. Break the cycle now.

My soul is dark with stormy riot,
directly traceable to diet.

SAMUEL HOFFENSTEIN

Diet HINT

To improve your mood without jeopardizing your waistline and your health, limit your sugar intake to no more than 10 percent of your calories (that means about 10 teaspoons if you are on a 2,000-calorie diet). To reach this goal, limit soda to one or two servings a week, since there are 8 to 10 teaspoons of sugar in one can; eat candy only as an occasional treat (there's another 5 to 8 teaspoons of sugar in each candy bar), and limit your cookie intake to a few small ones a week.

> No one can defeat us unless
> we first defeat ourselves.
>
> DWIGHT D. EISENHOWER

86 *If you're emotionally (and chemically) dependent on sugar to get you through your day, find healthy alternatives to foods high in processed sugar.*

When you eat something sweet, your blood sugar skyrockets, and you feel a rush of pleasure and well-being. Once the rush is gone, though, your blood sugar plummets, and you will probably feel worse than you did before. You may have a headache; you'll probably feel disheartened; and soon you'll crave another dose of sugar.

Break the cycle by turning from highly sugared snacks to more healthy carbohydrates, such as whole grains and starchy vegetables. Snack on half a wheat bagel topped with honey or a baked potato with a sprinkle of cheese, and you'll get the same emotional boost that you'd get from a candy bar—but without the blood-sugar drop that would follow the candy.

Diet FACT

We act as though our emotions are the concrete reality that shapes our world. But we need to remember that emotions like happiness and depression are actually the products of blood chemicals.

For instance, the chemical serotonin performs a variety of functions. High serotonin levels boost your mood, curb your food cravings, increase your pain tolerance, and help you sleep. Low levels of serotonin result in insomnia, depression, food cravings, increased sensitivity to pain, aggressive behavior, and poor body temperature regulation.

What we eat (and how much we exercise) has a powerful effect on serotonin.

Look at the Grand Canyon. It wasn't an earthquake that shaped it, but the gentle, persistent pressure of water.

ELSA WHITCOMB

87 *Reward yourself for your efforts.*

As you improve your eating and exercise habits, you will reap emotional as well as physical benefits. But you can't expect to see an overnight change in your emotions after you've made a change in your lifestyle. Dieting does not work the same as taking a pill; it will take two to three weeks of eating well before your body chemistry will adjust and you notice an improvement in your overall mood.

In the meantime, be extra nice to yourself in ways that don't involve food. Take a bubble bath. Buy yourself that book you've been wanting. Invest in scented lotions or a new nightgown. Reward yourself for having courage to begin this journey.

Change is hard.
So be kind to yourself while you're in the process.

RUBY TARR

> Just because we've carved a rut by taking the same path over and over, doesn't mean there aren't plenty of better paths we might choose to follow.
>
> LACY BROWN

88 *Learn new habits for handling sadness.*

Do you know the story about Pavlov and his dogs? Every time he fed his pooches, he also rang a bell. Pretty soon, the dogs, were drooling whenever a bell rang. They had learned to connect bells and food.

In a similar way, many of us have learned to crave desserts, breads, or other carbohydrate-loaded foods whenever we are tired, depressed, or anxious. These carbohydrate-rich snacks raise our serotonin levels and make us feel energized. Like Pavlov's dogs, who received food each time they heard a bell, we're rewarded each time we indulge our cravings. The food we eat increases our serotonin levels and makes us feel better.

But we can find other, healthier ways to lift our spirits.

I am an addict—a sugar addict.
I have turned to brownies and chocolate sundaes
when I should have turned to God.

ODETTE SCOTT

> Regret is an appalling waste of time.
> You can't build on it; it's good
> only for wallowing in.
>
> KATHERINE MANSFIELD

89 *Don't waste time feeling guilty.*

We already mentioned that guilt is a poor motivator for establishing an exercise routine. It's not a good reason to change the way you eat, either. Although healthy guilt based on reality may provide the initial impetus for change, ongoing guilt will only sap your strength. It is a negative emotion that does little good. After long enough, you will begin seeking a way to soothe the pain of bearing this heavy burden—and you may turn to food (even if overeating is the source of your guilt in the first place).

We have all fallen short of God's best. That's one reason why He sent His Son, so that Jesus could bear our guilt and we wouldn't have to anymore. Give your guilt to God. If it keeps coming back to haunt you, then, if need be, make a conscious decision to give it to Him every morning and every night. Let Him carry the load of your mistakes and failures. When He does, you'll find you can get on with your diet journey much more quickly.

All fall short of God's glorious standard.
Yet now God in his gracious kindness
declares us not guilty.

ROMANS 3:23–24 NLT

> No [woman's] life, even the happiest,
> is without its struggles and sacrifices.
>
> WILHELM VON HUMBOLDT

90 Don't expect to be happy all the time.

Sitcoms, TV commercials, and even the music industry all bombard us with the message that we ought to be happy. We've become brainwashed into believing that happiness is life's normal condition—and if we find ourselves unhappy, then we need only buy a product, fix a relationship, take a pill—or eat something—in order to magically restore our contentment.

Early generations, however, approached life much differently. They expected to endure hardship—and they understood that happiness is not always the benchmark of a healthy life.

God *does* want to give us His joy. But divine joy is not always the same thing as the emotion we call happiness. If we can learn to accept that our emotions will fluctuate—sometimes we will be happy, sometimes not—then we will be less inclined to automatically reach for food to soothe our sadness.

For what is our hope, our joy. . .
in which we will glory in the presence
of our Lord Jesus when he comes?

1 THESSALONIANS 2:19

> Obesity is a mental state,
> a disease brought on by boredom
> and disappointment. The way to get thin
> is to reestablish a purpose in life.
>
> CYRIL CONNOLLY

91 *Don't use food to counteract boredom. Find other interests.*

Sometimes we eat simply out of boredom, because we're not quite sure what else to do with ourselves. Eating becomes a form of self-stimulation.

If you find yourself turning to food to counter boredom, then you need to seek out other, healthier ways for breaking up life's monotony. Take up a hobby. Focus on another person's problem. Read your favorite magazine. Turn on the radio. Play with a child—or a pet. Find small, calorie-free passions to pursue each and every day.

92

Be aware of the connection between your hormonal cycle and your food cravings.

According to researchers at the Massachusetts Institute of Technology, women who experienced premenstrual stress also had cravings for carbohydrates. These women consumed as much as 87 percent more calories during the two weeks before their periods than they did during the rest of the month. Their sugar intake increased by as much as 20 teaspoons daily.

The researchers also found that these women had low serotonin levels during their two weeks of premenstrual symptoms. The women had learned to overeat carbohydrates in order to raise their serotonin—and improve their moods.

But it's another one of those self-defeating cycles. Other researchers at Texas A & M University discovered that if women removed sugar (and caffeine) from their diets, their symptoms of depression and fatigue disappeared. When they ate more complex carbohydrates instead (such as whole-grain pastas and breads), their premenstrual stress diminished.

When I think I need more sugar in my life—
I really need more God in my life.

LISA CURTIS

93 Wait fifteen minutes before giving in to a craving.

We're so used to thinking that our happiness depends on having what we want right now. But the next time you feel that your happiness will be incomplete without something sweet and fattening, trying telling yourself to simply wait for another fifteen minutes. During that time, you may find that your attention is diverted by something else. And you might find that your craving goes away by itself.

I know the price of success:
dedication, hard work, and an unremitting devotion
to the things you want to see happen.

FRANK LLOYD WRIGHT

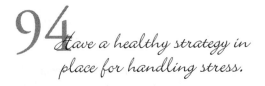

94 Have a healthy strategy in place for handling stress.

Stress is unavoidable. Sooner or later, circumstances bring to each of us our share of difficult situations. When that happens, our bodies' natural defense systems are weakened. Emotionally, we are prone to depression and anxiety. All too often, we turn to food for comfort.

When we are stressed, however, is the very time our bodies most need us to take care of them. A healthy strategy for handling stress includes these points:

Breakfast every day.
A high-nutrient, low-fat diet.
Limited alcohol.
Avoiding tobacco.
At least seven hours of sleep a night.
Daily exercise.
Less than ten hours of work a day.

193

Spending time with loved ones.
Laughing every day.
Making regular time for God throughout each day.

The art of living lies less in eliminating our troubles than in growing with them.

BERNARD M. BARUCH

That we might arrive at that region
of never-failing plenty, where
Thou feedest Israel for ever
with the food of truth.

AUGUSTINE

95 Tell yourself that God has given you everything you need.

Words have power—and the messages we tell ourselves shape our emotions. So watch your self-talk.

When I pay attention to the running dialogue inside my head, I often realize the many negative messages with which I bombard myself:

I have to eat that cookie.

A little won't hurt anything.

I've already blown my diet, so I might as well eat all I want.

I'll bet similar thoughts fill your head, too. Try replacing them with more positive self-talk:

God has given me all I truly need.

I am satisfied with the blessings God has given me.

I ate more than I wanted to, but God is offering me His forgiveness and strength.

If we believe that God has really and truly given us everything we need *right now*, we won't be as apt to turn to food for emotional comfort.

Enough is not only as good as a feast,
but is all that the greatest glutton can truly enjoy.

CHARLES SPURGEON

The Lord is my shepherd;
I have everything I need.

PSALM 23:1 NLT

> What is it that feeds thee? Joy.
>
> AUGUSTINE

96 *Don't make your diet the focus of your entire life.*

God wants our lives to be full—not narrow, stingy things. He wants us to experience the depth and breadth of the world He has created.

Don't become fixated on losing weight; don't make the decreasing numbers on the scales your only goal. If you do, you may become depressed, frustrated, or bored. Instead, dare to dream. Set yourself goals in other areas of your life. Invest in the world God has given you.

> Strange how one's thoughts turn to food
> when there is nothing else to think of.
>
> JOHN COLTON AND CLEMENCE RANDOLPH

Think—and think regularly every day.
An open mind is the best beauty parlor.

Fay Wray

97 Don't confuse love with food.

For most of us, ever since we were tiny babies, food and our mother's love were connected in our experience. No wonder then that as adults we still have food and love mixed up in our hearts. When we feel sad and lonely, a good meal (preferably one high in carbohydrates) reassures us.

Food may indeed be an expression of love. But love comes in many shapes and forms. And when you want to demonstrate love to yourself, you need to find other ways of expressing love.

It seems to me that our three basic needs,
for food and security and love,
are so mixed and mingled and entwined
that we cannot straightly think of one without the other.

M. F. K. Fisher

198

98 *Find healthy ways to express your feelings.*

As Christian women, we sometimes feel we should never be cross, never be fearful, never be anxious or angry or resentful. Those emotions just don't seem very spiritual. . .and so we deny that we even have them.

Maybe that's why so many of us are overweight. We're so used to denying ourselves in so many ways, especially emotionally—and food is the one outlet we allow ourselves. All our rage and despair and dread are soaked up by ice cream and potato chips and pastries.

Don't be afraid to own your emotions. Only then can you give them to God.

What you resist persists; what you accept lightens.

ANONYMOUS

Diet HINT

When you want to go on an eating binge, take time to sit down with your journal. Practice naming the emotions you're feeling along with the craving for food. By keeping track of your feelings in your journal (along with your food and exercise), you will begin to recognize what's really motivating your desire for food.

Remember, it's no sin to have emotions; God is only displeased when we allow our emotions to become destructive either to ourselves or others. Once you've identified your emotion, imagine yourself placing it in God's hands.

In matters of grace you need a daily supply. You have no store of strength. Day by day must you seek help from above. . . . Never go hungry while the daily bread of grace is on the table of mercy.

Charles Spurgeon

99 Rely on God for strength moment by moment.

Don't expect God to give you in one fell swoop the emotional stamina you need to get through the next year. . .or month. . .or week. . .or even day. Instead, learn to be in touch with Him every second. This doesn't mean you'll be engaged in conscious prayer every minute—but it does mean that your awareness of God is a constant presence in your life.

The difference between eating and overeating often lies in what you do with a single minute—the minute when you stop eating and remove yourself from the table before you start to overeat; the minute when you decide to walk instead of ride. If you start to stumble in that minute, simply reach out your hand to God for help.

Good habits are not made
on birthdays,
nor Christian character
at the new year.
The workshop of character
is everyday life.
The uneventful and common hour
is where the battle is lost or won.

MALTBIE D. BABCOCK

We should all know more, live nearer to God,
and grow in grace, if we were more alone.
Meditation chews the cud and extracts
the real nutriment from the mental
food gathered elsewhere.

CHARLES SPURGEON

100 *Make time to be alone.*

No matter how good our intentions, we all lose our way all too easily. For instance, as you read a book like this one, you may be filled with resolve to change your eating habits—but in the course of the busy week ahead, you may completely forget that resolution. The world's pressures and distractions drown out all other voices.

That's why we all need time in our busy schedules for moments alone with God. Those are the times we can meditate on His will for our lives. We can draw strength from His Word. We can take comfort from prayer.

And those quiet moments give us strength to face the noisy busy times.

A little with quiet is the only diet.

GEORGE HERBERT

I have esteemed the words of his mouth
more than my necessary food.

JOB 23:12 KJV

> Do I live on the manna
> which comes down from heaven?
> What is that manna but
> Jesus Christ Himself incarnate?
>
> CHARLES SPURGEON

101 *Feed on Jesus.*

When we're spiritually starved, we often reach for physical food instead.

When you get the urge to eat, ask yourself if you are really hungry—or are you eating to soothe some other hunger? Sometimes we try to use physical food to meet a spiritual need. No matter how much we eat, we will never be able to truly satisfy these hungers—and we are cheating ourselves of an opportunity for real satisfaction. We are nourishing our bodies, while we deprive our souls.

Instead of heading for the refrigerator, try reading a good book. . .listening to your favorite music. . .or praying. Don't starve your soul. And you may find that after you spend time with Jesus, your craving has disappeared.

Watch over your heart
with all diligence,
for from it flow
the springs of life.

PROVERBS 4:23 NAS